MIRACLES
OF
MILITARY
MEDICINE

MIRACLES
OF
MILITARY
MEDICINE

ALBERT Q. MAISEL

Essay Index Reprint Series

BOOKS FOR LIBRARIES PRESS
FREEPORT, NEW YORK

Copyright, 1943, by
Albert Q. Maisel

Reprinted 1972 by arrangement with
Hawthorn Books, Inc.

Library of Congress Cataloging in Publication Data

Maisel, Albert Q
    Miracles of military medicine.

    (Essay index reprint series)
    1. Medicine, Military. I. Title.
RC971.M35 1972   616.9'8023   70-167382
ISBN 0-8369-2561-0

PRINTED IN THE UNITED STATES OF AMERICA
BY
NEW WORLD BOOK MANUFACTURING CO., INC.
HALLANDALE, FLORIDA 33009

For

Dutsa and Merry

CONTENTS

INTRODUCTION   ix

I. SHOCK . . . THE EX-KILLER   3

II. "THAT SMELLY LITTLE SPANISH DOCTOR"   44

III. DOCTOR MOORHEAD'S SECRET WEAPON   74

IV. UNSEATING THE FOURTH HORSEMAN   90

V. NEW FACES FOR NEW MEN   115

VI. NO MORE TETANUS   137

VII. THE MINDSAVERS   163

VIII. THE JAPS GOT THE QUININE   182

IX. TAKING THE TERROR OUT OF WAR'S WORST WOUNDS   209

X. THE SULFA QUINTET   225

XI. THE NEW MAGIC OF LOCAL ANAESTHESIA   251

XII. FLYING DOCTORS   273

XIII. BLITZ MEDICINE FOR BLITZ WARFARE   312

XIV. WHEN SWORDS WILL BE SHEATHED   348

INTRODUCTION

THIS is a war of new weapons, far more accurate, far more pervasive, far more deadly than any that have ever been used before. In hundreds of books and thousands of articles, in every paper and over every radio, the power of these weapons has been broadcast and ballyhooed until even the youngest schoolboy can recite the lethal qualities of Zeros, Flying Fortresses, General Grants, Waltzing Mathildas, and Stormoviks. But there is another kind of new weapon that may play just as important a part in winning this war: a type of weapon that is little discussed and less well-known than any of our new planes and tanks. These are our new medical weapons, *the weapons that save lives.*

To a very substantial degree, the new tools of medicine and surgery have already gone far to counterbalance the greater destructive power of our modern war weapons. It is these new drugs, devices, and techniques which maintain the fighting strength of our troops at a higher level than ever before. These weapons are vital to the maintenance of morale and the will to fight in the face of mechanized destruction. In the final reckoning, these weapons will be responsible for the fact that tens and hundreds of thousands of men, who would have died in any previous war, won't die in this one.

Military medicine has kept pace with the development of war itself. It has, in fact, advanced so far within the last generation that the change has been converted from a quantitative to a qualitative one. During the last war, despite all the advances of the preceding hundred years, the men responsible for maintaining and restoring the health of armies were helpless against a score of scourges which today we can and do control and defeat. Disease, in a hundred different forms, killed millions of men, often before they reached their first battle. Infection of battle wounds carried off hundreds of thousands who today can be restored to full health. The lack of some of our newer drugs or techniques spelled a sentence of death for many tens of thousands and condemned others to lives of endless pain and incapacitation.

But today we have the sulfa drugs, we have bottled and dried blood, we have new pain-killers, new anaesthetics, new forms of treatment, new surgical procedures. We have the toxoids that are wiping out tetanus, the inoculations that end the menace of yellow fever. We have synthetic specifics against malaria without which our armies could not hope to fight in the tropics. Most important of all, we have developed to a high level of perfection the means for bringing these inventions to the individual soldier.

Only a few of these new developments have come to the attention of the general public. We all know something about the sulfa drugs because they are used in civil practice as well as in military medicine. We have had to learn something about dried blood plasma because we, the public at large, form the ultimate reservoir from whom the blood stream flows. But for the rest, most of the miracles of military medicine have been embalmed, as it were, in the specialized journals of the medical fraternity. This is not as strange as it may seem at first glance. Our physicians and surgeons have been too busy developing and applying their miracles to take time out to inform us of their work.

It has devolved therefore upon a layman to bring these stories to those whose interest in military medicine is personal rather than professional. Yet I have been most conscious of the pitfalls that beset the lay writer who ventures a popular discussion of medical subjects. While I have felt it important to bring out the hopeful aspects of these newer developments, I knew that I must at all costs avoid raising false or unjustified hopes. This problem I have attempted to solve by leaning upon the numerous medical men who were kind enough to help me with advice, analysis, and criticism. This aid is acknowledged, wherever possible, by references to individuals at appropriate places in the text.

But grateful acknowledgment is due to a number of military and medical men, who despite the burden of their war duties have taken much time and great pains to guide and correct my writing or to open to me sources of information not ordinarily available to the layman.

I want particularly to express my appreciation to Colonel Edgar Erskine Hume and Lieutenant Herbert S. Stare for information on the work of the Medical Field Service School at Carlisle, Pa. Major Charles H. Wilson, Director of the Department of Field Medicine and Surgery at Carlisle, has been most helpful in acquainting me with many of the newer devices and drugs used in surgical work in the field. Dr. John J. Moorhead, Professor of Traumatic Surgery at Post Graduate Hospital Medical School, has not only supplied much information on medical problems met at Pearl Harbor but has served to guide my thinking in respect to many another problem as well. Dr. Justus Rice, Medical Director of the Winthrop Chemical Company, has made available to me his extensive bibliographies without which the chapter on the fight against malaria could not have been written.

Captain Julian J. Fried and Lt. Donald Weisman, both in their capacity as personal friends and as members of the Medical Corps of the Army, have helped me over innumerable hurdles, corrected me on matters of fact and guided me on questions of viewpoint. For much of the information on medical and military developments and experiments carried on in Russia, I am indebted to A. Timofeev, Third Secretary of the Embassy of the Soviet Union, who has made available to me numerous reports on Soviet military medicine. Dr. Edward Barsky has provided me with invaluable information on military-medical developments, based upon his experience and observation as a surgeon with the Republican Army during the Civil War in Spain.

To numerous others, with whom I have not had the pleasure of face-to-face contact, but who have contributed to this work either through personal communications or through their writings, grateful acknowledgment is due. Roscoe Clarke, F.R.C.S., First Assistant in Surgery at the British Postgraduate Medical School, first pointed me towards some of the newer developments in Russian Medicine. Dr. Winnett Orr, Chief Surgeon of the Nebraska Orthopedic Hospital, whose quarter-century fight for the Closed Plaster Method of treating fractures has now been everywhere acclaimed where once it met only skepticism, first put me on the track of Dr. José Trueta, the "smelly little Spanish doctor" of Chapter II. The chapter on burn therapy, "Unseating the Fourth Horseman," could not have been written but for the painstaking research and catholic knowledge of Dr. Henry N. Harkins, Associate Surgeon of the Henry Ford Hospital of Detroit. The same is true of the chapter, "Flying Doctors," which owes much, in detail and in viewpoint, to Major Henry G. Armstrong, one of the outstanding pioneers of aviation medicine.

The hundreds of others who, in one way or another, have made this book possible, will, I know, forgive those instances in which I have borrowed their thoughts and told of their discoveries without individual credit.

While reliance upon the advice of medical men may serve to insure this work against errors of fact and misinterpretations of the relative importance of facts, it cannot protect any book against the progress of medicine itself. Military medicine is advancing at so rapid a pace that some of the facts and figures I have cited may become out of date even before this volume leaves the presses. It is comforting to know that, should this happen, the change will undoubtedly be one for the better. It is not every author who can feel as certain as I do that the sequel to his writings will be prepared for him, even as he writes. More power then to the medical men of our armed forces and those of our allies. May they speedily make obsolete even my most optimistic reports on their work.

ALBERT Q. MAISEL

MIRACLES
OF
MILITARY
MEDICINE

Chapter I

SHOCK . . . THE EX-KILLER

THE squad tumbled back into the water-logged trench one by one. The night's reconnaissance was over and the young lieutenant breathed a sigh of relief as he rolled after his men into the safety that lay behind the parapet.

"Four hours out in that muck and we haven't had a single scratch. Our luck was sure with us tonight," he thought as he wrapped his half-frozen hands around the steaming tin cup of coffee which someone had placed in them. Just one thing left to do and then they could all tumble into the dugout for five hours of exhausted sleep.

From force of habit he whispered, "At ease, men," as he crawled past the crouching bodies of his mud-stained crew. It wasn't an order, he knew, for not one of them could have stood at attention even for General Haig himself. But the men liked it better if you showed them you thought about such things and Lieutenant Crofts knew, intuitively, how to keep his men plugging together as a unit.

The field telephone was in a little box of a dugout, a sort of cave in the trench wall about thirty paces off. Crofts lifted the instrument and turned the crank. During that long moment of waiting for the operator back at headquarters to wake up, he began to realize how tired he really was. When the thin, calm voice at the other end said, "Ready here," he had to shake himself back to consciousness before he could make his report.

Then he made for the dugout. He entered quietly, remembering the position of every bunk and carefully avoiding the gear which he knew would be piled at the center of the room. He made his bunk, the one behind the table at the rear, without a sound and had just started to roll over when a voice said, "Beg pardon, sir?"

"Yes, who is it?"

"Banting, sir."

"Well, tumble in, Banting."

"But, sir, there's a man missing."

Crofts shook his head again, hard this time. Then he yelled, "Lights on." A match flared and there stood Banting, lighting the oil lamp. In its growing glow he counted off the mud-stained faces. Grumman, Myers, Jones, Scudder, Borden, Loeb . . . Peters? Banting was right. Peters, the green kid they had sent him last week to replace Cutler, Peters was missing.

The men realized it just about the same second.

Someone dashed out into the trench. The rest waited in silence. Then he came back, shaking his head. "His gun's not in the rack, sir."

One after the other, Indian file, they followed Crofts back to the parapet. Outside, it was still, except when the breeze brought the sound of a distant shell from over the hills to the left. Ears cocked, they listened. Then Myers nudged him. "Over there, to the left, sir. I just heard him."

Again they listened. Nothing.

Then again, a thin, faint sound—the sort of sound you never hear except during the darkest part of the night.

"That's him," Crofts whispered. "I'll need one man."

Then he lifted himself over the edge of the trench and started to crawl. He knew, as he inched forward, that all seven of them had followed him. He knew that he couldn't have ordered them back, so he didn't try. Just kept on crawling.

They found Peters only a hundred yards out. He'd never even got beyond their own wire.

Crofts whispered, "Where'd it get you?"

"My leg, below the knee. I'd have made it crawling, sir. You needn't have come."

"Sure, sure," Crofts answered. "But we're here now, so relax."

Three of them took off their shirts and they made a sort of cradle out of them. Then they rolled Peters onto it and started dragging him back. Twice they thought a Jerry had spotted them, when there was some stirring across the wire. But luck was still with them and they made it, just as the sky began to lighten behind them.

When they got Peters into the trench and examined his wound, it looked better than they had expected. A straight puncture. A lot of blood lost but no bones broken. They all cheered up a bit then and when Peters asked for a cigarette, they all lit up.

"I won't send for a replacement, Peters," Crofts said. "They'll have you back here in a week."

But Crofts was worried. More than he wanted to let on. The kid could have lost a whale of a lot of blood in five hours. His skin was cold, clammily cold. His breathing was fast.

Then the stretcher-bearers came up the communications trench and they lifted Peters onto the pallet. Crofts thought of giving the kid his odds and ends. They lay scattered on his bunk, a picture, a book, his razor. Then he decided not to. He handed Peters a pack of butts instead and they carried him off.

It was three days before the company was relieved and another day before Crofts could get time off himself. Then he made for the Divisional Hospital.

Peters wasn't there. Yes, they had brought him in. He'd been doing well, they had thought, but he died of shock before they could get him to the operating table. The doctor said it in such a matter-of-fact way that Crofts forgot his rank as he snapped, "What the hell do you mean, shock?"

The doctor began to get angry . . . then, in a split second, he subsided.

"I wish I knew what we meant, son. I wish we all knew what we meant. All we know about shock is that we lose a lot of good men who should never die from their wounds alone. Something happens to their systems. Peters lost a lot of blood but sometimes they die of shock even though there is no blood loss. It just comes over them a few hours after they're injured. Their blood pressure falls, their pulses get small and rapid, their temperature drops, their skin becomes cold, they breathe faster and faster—and then they either snap out of it or they—die. Just like that."

"But, doctor, isn't there anything that can be done about it? After all—"

"Yes, lieutenant, there are a few things we've learned. We keep them warm, use hot blankets, give them hot drinks. It helps. Might have helped your lad Peters, if we'd gotten him sooner. Or if he'd lasted till we could have given him a blood transfusion . . . that sometimes helps, too."

That was shock in 1917: shock the great killer. Something doctors had known since first wars were fought, and something they still knew practically nothing about.

Most of us have experienced shock, in mild form, many times during our lives.

Shock evidences itself in the faintness you feel after —sometimes *hours* after—a strong emotional experience.

Shock was what made you grow cold and clammy the time you took that unexpected punch just below the ribs.

It was shock that made you grow pale and cold the time you had that nose bleed you couldn't stop.

And it was to avoid shock that the dentist made you stay in his office for nearly an hour after he took your tooth out that cold, rainy day.

"Well, now," you say, "that sounds annoying enough, but really not so very terrible. Surely it can't be that slight reaction that kills men like Private Peters, men who have those minor kinds of wounds that doctors know just how to deal with." Yet it *is* the same thing, differing only in degree.

The trouble with telling about it is that it is just as hard to describe as your feeling of faintness. Doctors, in fact, have been troubled with its description and— even more—with its mechanism for generations. Upon one thing, however, they are all agreed. In the presence of shock there is a marked decrease in the amount of circulating blood in the system of veins and arteries.

How simple the whole problem of understanding shock (but not necessarily the problem of treating it) would be, if all cases were as simple as an uncomplicated hemorrhage. Suppose we cut an artery and blood flows out, lots of blood. Since we are subtracting blood from a closed system, you can see why the flow of blood to any part of the system is reduced. And why the blood pressure falls.

But what about an internal hemorrhage? Well, that is a bit more complicated. Yet we still have blood subtracted from the system of veins and arteries. In fact, doctors sometimes deduce the fact of hemorrhage by the presence of an otherwise unaccountable state of shock, as in the case of persons with peptic ulcers who grow faint from loss of blood (i.e., from shock) although that loss occurs *within* the body.

So far, it seems somewhat simple. The way to overcome shock would seem to be by the administration of a compensating amount of blood, or some substitute, to replace the blood lost by hemorrhage. That should do the trick and, in fact, it does do the trick if loss of blood, whole blood, is the principal cause of the shocked state.

However, the body's circulatory system is not by any means as simple as, let us say, the cooling system of your car. Nor is the blood as simple a fluid as the water you put into your car's radiator. And these two indescribably complicated facts make themselves painfully apparent to every doctor who tries to treat shock cases—particularly under the difficult conditions of wartime. All sorts of difficulties present themselves to the physician and every time he thinks he has climbed over one of them, another seems to pop up to give him renewed troubles.

Take the seemingly simple matter of blood transfusion. I say, "seemingly simple," because it has the simplicity of something we have all accepted as almost a commonplace. It's simple in the same sense that an auto engine is simple. Most of us haven't any too clear an idea of exactly how the engine works, but we know well enough how to operate it, how to make it start and stop.

If you stop to think of it, about all most of us know about blood transfusion is what we've picked up from watching Paul Muni and Lew Ayres do it in the movies.

However, before Dr. Kildare could use a blood transfusion to save his sweetheart's life, hundreds and hundreds of doctors had to piece together our knowledge of the difficult procedure over many decades. The *idea* of transfusion is an old one that springs up again and again in medical history. But the practical application of that idea was one long history of failures until 1900.

The trouble was that doctors, probably in reaction against the superstitions that lent all sorts of mystical properties to blood, had until then looked upon all blood—and particularly all human blood—as interchangeable. Two or three or four times running, they would have amazingly successful results from attempted transfusions. Then, the next time they tried it, for some strange and incomprehensible reason, the transfusion would kill the patient.

Whereupon the doctor would find himself charged with malpractice, witchcraft, or murder. All of which had, shall we say, a tendency to discourage further experimentation.

Then, in 1900, the Viennese doctor, Landsteiner, demonstrated the presence of agglutinating substances in human blood. The next year he divided blood into three groups and showed how the mixing of these groups caused the strange reactions that had so confounded the earlier experimenters.

After that, it was easy sailing.

Within a year others showed that there were really four blood groups and still others worked out the practical matter of identifying or "typing" these groups so that doctors could be sure that they gave the right kind of blood to the patient.

In order to get a better picture of just what the doctors did discover, let's take a look at a little chart:

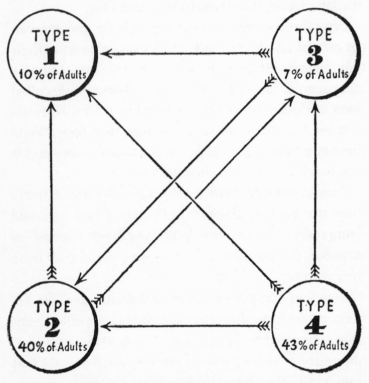

About ten per cent of all adults have blood of type one. These people may give blood only to their own type group. If their blood is transfused to any recipients outside of their group, agglutination reactions occur and possibly death. But they can receive blood from all four groups, their own and the other three. So they are called universal recipients.

Type two includes about forty per cent of all adults. They can give blood to types one and three. And they can take blood from types three and four.

Type three is the smallest group, only about seven per cent of adults. (Infants don't usually develop their type characteristics until they are from nine months to a year old. Of course, infants are almost never called upon to donate blood, but it is convenient sometimes to know that they can take any type of blood.) Type three can take blood from types two and four; and it can give blood to types one and two.

Finally, we have type four, numbering about forty-three per cent of all adults. These are the universal donors, able to give blood to all four types, themselves included. But they are able to receive blood only from their own type.

Now you can see why, before Landsteiner, the experimenters in transfusion ran into such troubles. Suppose they tried to give blood to a type four patient. Since fifty-seven per cent of all people fall outside that type group, the chances were a little better than even that they would strike a donor unsuited to their patient.

With the other groups they had a better statistical chance. With type three, all but ten per cent of possible donors are theoretically acceptable. With type two, the same condition is true. And with type one, no trouble, as far as agglutination is concerned, was to be anticipated.

Once the problem of typing was largely eliminated, or at least understood, progress in transfusion techniques was rapid. The principal remaining difficulty lay in the fact that the blood tended to coagulate in the transfusing apparatus.

The earliest attempts to solve this problem sought to eliminate the apparatus itself. Doctors invented ingenious little devices which permitted them to slip a vein through a little pipe, cuff it back over the pipe, and then slip the donor's artery over the cuffed vein. Thus the blood never touched anything but human "blood pipes." Yet this method had two unfavorable features. For one thing it involved the sacrifice of an artery on the part of the donor. For another, it made impossible the accurate measurement of the amount of blood transfused.

Both of these difficulties were overcome shortly by the introduction of devices that pumped the blood, rapidly, from the donor's artery into the recipient's veins—so rapidly as to overcome a large part of the tendency towards coagulation. And finally, in 1914, anti-coagulation substances were introduced which virtually eliminated the problem. The best of these, and still used today, is citrate.

Thus, just as the first World War began, medicine was armed with one of its greatest life-saving tools, the ability to transfuse blood on a regular, predictable, controllable basis. And the doctors used it—used it wherever they possibly could.

But even so, blood transfusion as practiced in the first World War had very definite limitations. The first of these was the simple fact that you had to bring your donor and your recipient into direct contact or at least you had to put them simultaneously in the same building. For the techniques they then had didn't include either the preservation or the transportation of the donor's blood.

That, if you remember, was one of the main reasons why Private Peters died. He just didn't last long enough to get far enough back from the front lines to receive a transfusion. For every one of the hundreds of thousands who were saved by transfusion during the last war, at least two others were in Private Peters' class.

After 1918 doctors met the same sort of problem in civil practice. Time and time again you couldn't get a suitable donor to the patient in time, particularly when you practiced in some out-of-the-way village. You tried using volunteers, but even then, you needed just the right type and the process of typing was a time-consuming one.

But the worst of it was when some disaster occurred, some earthquake or great fire or flood. Then, prepare as you would for it, you found yourself with more patients than available donors. And that thrust upon the doctors the hateful task of rationing life when they knew they didn't have enough to go around.

The man who first licked that problem was S. S. Yudin, Chief of the Surgical Clinic of the Central Emergency Hospital in Moscow. Dr. Yudin and his associates did something that other doctors, in other countries, had perhaps whispered about, as a possibility, but had never quite dared to try.

He used cadaver blood—blood drawn from the veins of persons who had died.

In perhaps no other country could a physician have dared this experiment. The idea would have proved too revolting to large groups, and very powerful groups, of people. In most countries, doctors must respect these sensibilities, no matter how much they may conflict with the cold logic of science. For that matter, Yudin, too, might have run into a storm of protest, had not the obvious success of his experiments provided the most tangible support for his position.

For, as against the few dead persons drained of their blood—and remember, drained after death which would have occurred in any event—against these few, Yudin produced, in 1936, over nine hundred persons who had been pulled back to life by his method.

Nor had Yudin tried his experiments without the firm support of earlier work upon which to base his hopes for success. For Soviet doctors had been working on the problem for at least eight years. By 1932, two investigators, Skundina and Berenboim, were able to report substantial successes in transfusion of blood from dogs, which had died a few hours before, into other test dogs. These experiments demonstrated that when cadavers were preserved at a temperature of one or two degrees above zero, the blood in the cadaver vessels preserved its living properties for six or seven hours.

By 1935, Skundina, working with Rosakov and Ginsberg, was able to report on what happened to blood in the hours after human death. And this report posed a mystery which has not been solved to this day; but a most convenient mystery, nevertheless. When cadaver blood was secured following rapid death, usually from accident, it rapidly coagulated. But strangely, within any time from a half hour to two hours, the coagulated blood became fluid again and thereafter would not coagulate. At first these researchers spent much time hunting for an explanation of this unexpected reversal of the coagulation process.

Then one of them—their published records fail to indicate which one—began to look beyond the mystery to its implications. Suddenly they realized that they had stumbled upon a phenomenon that might solve the whole problem of adjusting supply to demand, that might make transfusable blood available anywhere, at any time and in any quantity. For this blood could be preserved in its fluid state, indefinitely, without the addition of an anti-coagulant.

That was when Yudin came into the picture. Dr. Yudin and his co-workers, like physicians the world over, had long been troubled by the difficulty of getting blood donors in emergencies. You can well understand why they would be impelled to brush aside a hesitancy over religious or traditional scruples when suddenly the possibility opened up to them of saving life by eliminating delays with donors.

Here was blood, life-giving blood, of no further use to the corpse which yielded it—yet capable of saving the lives of others.

Far from feeling that there might be anything repugnant in the procedure, these workers might well maintain that now, even the dead, might give one last great service to their fellow men, a service quite as great as any they had given in their lifetimes.

It obviously wasn't a question of morals. The moral weight was all on the side of using the blood. But would it work?

Well, it had worked on the lower animals.

It had worked time and again on dogs.

So they turned to their patients and asked them if they would take a gambler's chance for science. They told them exactly how large, and exactly how small, the chance was.

Some, knowing that blood from living, human donors was available, chose not to take the chance. But others, who knew that some day soon blood from living donors might not be available for other people sick as they were, took the chance.

And these recovered. The preserved cadaver blood coursed through their veins just as Yudin had predicted it would. No complications ensued. No reactions. Death had fought back death.

Yet, after they were all through, these Russian doctors found that they had not done quite what they had set out to do. Their battle with tradition and superstition turned out to be unnecessary in most civil and—up to now—most military practice. Their own experiments made the use of cadaver blood unnecessary. They had, in the very process of their work, invented the blood bank. They had learned how to store blood. Not for a half hour, during the process of transfusion. But for days.

Other doctors, in countries where the use of cadaver blood might have met with stern opposition, were quick to see the implications of this phase of the Russian experiments. Throughout the world, doctors began to think of blood reservoirs, banks of stored blood that would tide them over a sudden peak in demand.

The idea burst upon the medical world with such suddenness that the records are not quite clear as to when and where the first blood bank was started.

But there is some fairly general agreement that the first bank put into systematic operation was at the Cook County Hospital in Chicago. Not that precedence matters too much, for others followed in quick succession wherever in the world doctors were faced with the pressing need for quick transfusions. Which means practically everywhere.

The doctors reasoned somewhat like this: Without storage, we must first decide that a transfusion is needed. Then we must secure a donor, easy enough at times but often devilishly difficult. We must bring the donor to the patient, and that takes time. If he isn't a professional, we must type him, and that takes more time. If he turns out to be acceptable as to type, we must still make sure that he isn't carrying some transmittable disease in his blood stream. And after all that, we must waste more time setting up our transfusion apparatus and draining the donor's blood into our patient's system.

All too often, the doctors knew from bitter experience, the patient couldn't wait that long. Even if he survived through all the waiting, the delay still had its price in lowered resistance, tissue damage, shock and suffering.

But suppose we do all these things before we actually need the blood. Before Johnny gets hit by an auto. Before Tom falls from a scaffold. Before Mabel's operation takes its toll in blood loss. Suppose we tap our donors on a regular schedule, under the finest laboratory conditions. We take our time in typing and testing. Suppose we deposit this blood in our bank, as if it were so much money, the money of life.

Then when we need it, we draw a draft on our bank. Out comes a bottle of the precious fluid, wherever we need it, whenever we need it. And all the Johnnies and Toms and Mabels don't have to wait and die for the lack of blood.

Simple, isn't it?

Like all miracles, it's simple when you've learned the trick. Here, the trick was not some single operation —some individual wonder of science. It was rather the sum of an almost infinite series of small discoveries, of additions to technique, of recorded experiences, that together grew and multiplied until, all at once, all the basic essentials of blood preservation were present and all that remained was for someone to put them together, to use them all at once.

That is why, no doubt, the blood bank has made such phenomenal progress since 1936. In civil life, at least, it represents the answer not just to a single problem, but to a score of related problems. It transforms blood transfusion from a tripartite miracle of co-operation between one donor, one patient, and one doctor into a multiple miracle in which hundreds of donors and doctors, widely separated in time and, if need be, in space, cooperate to meet the need of recipients even before their need has arisen.

It is an exceedingly complicated miracle. The technique of operation of a blood bank is one constant fight to preserve the blood, in all its life-giving qualities, until the draft is presented and the blood is drawn from the bank. These precautions start with donor selection, as in ordinary transfusion. Once the blood is secured, it must be sealed against every form of contamination for all the days it stays on deposit. Finally it must be turned over, in perfect condition, to the patient who needs it.

Naturally, these problems increase manyfold under wartime conditions. Before the time of test came there were many who doubted that blood banks could be used by armies in the field. As in so many other respects, the Civil War in Spain provided the testing ground and proved these fears to be largely false.

In Spain the first mass use of the blood bank under wartime conditions was attempted and successfully carried through. Could blood be safely transported up towards the front lines? The Spaniards, and their international medical helpers, proved that it could. Could the transfusions be safely administered by orderlies, if properly trained? Again Spain answered the question and proved that, in a mass emergency, there are never, have never been, enough doctors at any one place. If we free them from one task, we free them to do another, perhaps more important part of their work.

No wonder, then, that the British, when their time came, turned to their own doctors who had had experience in Spain. For more than ever, in air-raid casualties, are transfusions necessary. In Spain it had been found that at least ten per cent of air-raid victims required transfusion. In the vastly greater carnage that fell on London, Bristol, Coventry, and a score of other British cities, this ten per cent would have taxed and overtaxed any system of direct transfusion that could have been set up.

With blood banks the British, as they put it, "did quite nicely." Except at the very beginning, when some of the rough edges were still to be brushed from the technique, there was never a time in England when blood transfusions presented the major problem to air-raid workers.

For all that, the blood bank didn't solve the military transfusion problem. At least two more major difficulties remained. Luckily, the solution of the first of these involved, in great measure, the solution of the second. Both today have been solved, thoroughly and decisively, and just barely in time.

Before the doctors could make further progress they had to stop thinking of blood as a single, homogeneous substance. Instead they had to look into the various components of blood and find out the functions and nature of each.

When they did that, they found that blood consists of the red and white blood cells carried in a fluid material which they called plasma. The red cells pick up oxygen in the lungs and carry it to the organs and tissues. But they carry it only when the plasma is there, in sufficient quantity to maintain circulation and, moreover, to maintain transfer of oxygen from the red cells to the tissues and organs. The blood cells carry away the waste product of the tissues, carbon dioxide, also only when the plasma is there in proper quantity to permit adequate circulation and adequate functioning.

With a simple hemorrhage—if we can consider it as just so much leakage of blood from the body—it is whole blood that is being lost. The balance between the blood cells and the blood plasma doesn't change. Hence the problem is the relatively simple one of re-placing like with like, blood with blood.

But in "wound shock" and "burn shock" the process is far more complicated. The actual loss of blood may be very slight. In the case of burns, there may be no blood lost from the body at all. But substantial quan-tities of plasma may be lost, leaking through the capil-lary walls that usually hold against leakage, and escap-ing into the tissues. When this occurs, the blood goes out of balance and a vicious circle leading towards death is set into operation. The impact of a bullet, the tearing of flesh by a missile, the burning of a flame— all these may cause a lowering of the normal resistance of the capillaries to the passage of plasma through their membrane-like walls. When this happens our cycle begins.

Less fluid is available for return through the veins. Less reaches the heart. And the heart, in turn, pumps less into the arteries. Doctors can note this, for blood pressure falls, one of the surest signs of the oncoming of shock.

The reduced blood flow leads to asphyxia of the tissues. They suffocate for lack of blood-borne oxygen. They cannot get rid of their carbon-dioxide wastes. This, in turn, brings on further dilatation of the capillaries, in an attempt to compensate for the reduction in flow. But now more fluid passes through the capillary membranes. The red blood cells, which do not pass through, become more concentrated. The thicker blood flows still more slowly back to the heart. The vicious circle is in full swing.

The process goes on and on, until the victim dies, unless, somehow, you successfully interfere with it. If it hasn't proceeded too far, whole blood may be used. This would restore the plasma content to normal, although it would bring the red-cell content above normal. Up to a point the body could take care of that, provided sufficient plasma protein was replaced to maintain blood circulation and the feeding of oxygen to the tissues. If that can be achieved, the capillaries will gradually recover, dilatation will disappear, and the system will swing back into its former balance.

But suppose the loss of fluid has been great. Then no amount of whole blood which might be introduced could bring the system back into even approximate balance. I can think of no better way of illustrating the problem than by citing the example of a summer camp, filled with fifty young men and fifty young women. Everyone is, of course, happy, for the system is in perfect balance.

But if we take away thirty of the men, we throw the whole set-up out of kilter. For now we have only twenty youths to maintain "circulation" among fifty females.

Now suppose the owner of the camp tried to balance things by introducing thirty new people in the form of fifteen married couples. Obviously, he will not have begun to restore balance by such tactics. In fact the only thing that will restore balance would be another thirty or so of young men. Unless they are provided, all the girls will wither away for lack of "circulation" and the camp will go out of operation.

I hope you won't consider this parallel flippant, because that is exactly the problem that must be solved when we propose to treat traumatic shock caused by wounds or burns. Having lost plasma from the blood tree, we must restore plasma if we are to re-establish the balance that alone can break the vicious circle of shock.

Doctors discovered this fact a long time ago. But having no means of preserving blood, such as the blood bank, they had little or no experience with plasma. They therefore sought blood substitutes, fluids that would restore blood circulation by replacing the fluid losses that lead to shock.

A whole host of solutions imitating blood were developed. One of the most widely used during the last war was gum acacia. At that time it was heralded as a perfect blood substitute. But later experimentation showed it to have a number of disadvantages and even distinct dangers associated with its use. Acacia may induce serious liver damage. It may interfere with the oxygen-interchanging action of the red blood cells. It may cause conglutination of the red cells, blocking the smaller capillaries, and it may be followed by severe and sometimes fatal reactions.

But acacia, as well as saline solutions and other fluids, did have a favorable temporary effect. They restored blood volume and thus broke the vicious circle. Their main drawback was that, unlike plasma, they were quickly lost from the blood stream and then the whole process started over again, often aggravated in form.

Once doctors had their blood banks, however, they

found plasma practically forcing itself upon them. For after the whole blood had stood in the bank for some days, it separated. The cells dropped to the bottom, and the plasma, or most of it, stood on top. After the safe period for use of whole blood had passed, the doctors could just as easily rescue the plasma as throw it away. Naturally, they experimented extensively with the fluid.

From there on, progress was rapıa, for to the experts the need for plasma was a crying one. Ironically enough, they had tried to invent something to replace plasma and, now, plasma replaced their inventions.

You will remember that we spoke of *two* major military transfusion difficulties that remained even after the invention of the blood-bank technique. The first of these, the need for a replacement fluid other than whole blood, was solved by the separation of plasma from the blood. At the same time, the discovery and development of the plasma-using technique served to solve the second problem, that of bringing the transfusion up to the soldier instead of bringing the wounded to the transfusion.

The first great advantage of plasma over blood, from a military point of view, is the fact that no donor-typing is necessary. Since the antagonistic substances that cause reactions when blood types are mixed occur in the blood cells rather than in the plasma, the minute we separate our plasma we eliminate the problem of typing.

Secondly, plasma may be stored for months without significant alteration, as long as it is kept cool. No need, when you use plasma, to worry about replacing the blood in the bank as you withdraw it. True eventually the plasma bank must be replenished just as the blood bank, but the ability to preserve plasma over long periods gives much more leeway.

. Moreover, a lot of our plasma can be obtained as a waste product of our regular blood banks. That pint you donated may first rest in a local bank as whole blood until its period of usefulness has passed. Then, having served its function as part of the banked reserve, it can go on to serve again, in the form of blood plasma.

Finally, we have the fact that plasma is easily transported and easily administered. It can therefore be used right up at the front lines, if necessary.

Thus, for military purposes, plasma represents an even greater advance than did blood transfusion itself during the last war.

This may seem like a contradiction, for the use of plasma is, you will say, merely an extension of the transfusion technique. If you were talking about civil use, you might be right or partially right. But in military medicine, the time element is the all-important factor in wound treatment. Mortality almost invariably increases as the square of the time between wounding and treatment. If we move our transfusion technique up halfway to the front lines, we give our soldiers not twice as good a chance of surviving a wound, we increase their chances four times.

With plasma, the transfusion process moves right into the front lines. The time element is cut not to half but to some tiny fraction, one-tenth or one-twentieth of the time that formerly must have elapsed before the soldier could be brought to the donor. Thus shock is stopped before it can get started.

The full import of this advance can only be appreciated when we remember that the bulk of the wounded, who formerly died in transport between the first-aid post and the casualty clearing station, did not die of their wounds at all. On the contrary, they died of shock or of hemorrhage and the shock attendant thereto.

Yet even fluid plasma does not represent the last word in shock therapy. For the law of the acceleration of invention has been busily at work.

Hundreds of years passed, from the time man first tried transfusion of blood until the day when the discovery of blood types laid the basis for modern transfusion practices.

It took fifteen more years before the technique of transfusion was developed to the point where it could be applied on a wide enough scale to be a factor in military medicine.

It took a full additional generation before the blood bank was invented, making it unnecessary to get the patient to the donor and solving much of the time and transport difficulties that formerly limited the usefulness of transfusion.

It took another five years for plasma therapy to come into general use, further cutting the time lag and solving the problems of fluid replacement.

But it took only one additional year for the last—and perhaps greatest—step in anti-shock work. That step is represented by the development of dried plasma. Here again, it is difficult to lay credit for the work at any single man's doorstep. For the need was long foreseen and many experimenters have been at work on a variety of processes for some time.

Essentially, all these processes have a common aim. By removing the water content of plasma, they reduce the essential proteins to a dry, yellow powder. This powder can be preserved, in vacuum, indefinitely and it can be restored or reconstituted, with all its properties unchanged, simply by restoring the water content through the addition of distilled water.

Its advantages over liquid plasma are quite as great as those of the liquid over whole blood. First we have greater stability. While the liquid plasma can be preserved for some time at room temperature (especially if kept in the dark), storage under refrigeration is preferable. But dried plasma, in vacuum containers, is stable indefinitely at room temperature, even in tropical climates.

Secondly, we have a further great reduction in bulk. Dried plasma takes less than eight per cent of the space of fluid plasma. It can be carried in a tiny kit by first-aid men. Blood transfusions can, at last, move right up to the firing line, if need be.

A third advantage is found in increased transportability. Not only is this due to the reduction in bulk, but also to the immunity from alteration which the dried product enjoys. While whole blood or plasma may deteriorate from lack of refrigeration, agitation, or any of the other hazards of transit, the dried product is as stable as hard-tack.

Yet all these advantages pale before a final, all-important property of dried or desiccated plasma. Whole blood and liquid plasma must be administered pretty much as nature made them. But dried plasma may be given in any desired concentration simply by cutting the amount of water to be added to the plasma powder. The administration of concentrated plasma is of particular importance when the injury is of such a nature as to cause substantial fluid loss through the capillaries into the tissues. For here the restoration of proteins to the blood stream can literally reverse the process. As the protein content of the blood mounts, osmotic pressure, which previously forced more and more fluid *out* of the blood vessels into the surrounding tissues, is now turned about and the flow starts in the opposite direction.

Obviously, when this is the aim—as, for instance, where swelling is occurring because of the transfer of blood fluids to the tissues—concentration of plasma provides great advantages. For the concentrated product affords a speedy rise in the protein content of the blood. And instead of transfusing water into the blood system, we draw it back into the system by the magnet of osmotic pressure—drawing it out of the tissues where it is causing swelling and inviting infection.

So, at last, with the development of dried plasma came a method of transfusion that could fight shock to a standstill. And it came just in time.

No greater tribute can be paid the medical fraternity than to put on record the simple fact that our medical rearmament not only kept pace with our war industries during the period of "neutrality," but actually outstripped every other phase of our war preparation. When Tojo struck at Pearl Harbor, the admirals and generals may have been half asleep, but the doctors, at least, were ready.

How that state of readiness was achieved is a story of heroic proportions and one which demonstrates that Lend-Lease has not, by any means, been a one-way street. For every boy that was saved at Pearl Harbor and Bataan—and for every one who will yet be saved on a hundred more battlefields—we will owe a debt to the doctors of America who could not stand idly by while their British comrades needed aid during the darkest days of 1940.

For instance, there was Dr. John Scudder, who for some years had been doing research work on plasma at New York's Presbyterian Hospital. In May and June, 1940, Dr. Scudder, like the rest of us, read with dismay the daily record of the Nazis' progress through the Low Countries and France. We, as laymen, could see only horror in the tales of stukas bombing the refugee-choked roads. But to Scudder each news dispatch spelled not only horror but opportunity. Here was something a physician could get a grip on. Here was a real need for the techniques he had worked on in the quiet of his laboratory.

One night early in June, Scudder sat down with his old friend and associate, John Bush. Both men had spent years working together, Bush as President of the Blood Transfusion Association, Scudder as one of the most active researchers in the field. As Scudder broached the plan that had been germinating in his mind, he found no opposition from Bush. For how could anyone oppose the idea of saving life if he had already given years of his own life to that very idea?

The plan was simple in the extreme. Bush's Association would mobilize the funds, the technical resources, and the voluntary aid of New York's doctors and hospitals. Together this well-equipped medical army would be able to gather the voluntary blood donations of New York's people. After processing the blood, they would ship it to England and—they still hoped—to France, where the shattered blood services of smashed armies could not possibly keep up with the mounting, skyrocketing needs.

On June 12, 1940, Bush called a joint meeting of the Association's Trustees and Board of Medical Control. In a single room, in the great Academy of Medicine, there met the city's leading specialists in blood transfusion as well as experts of the Army and Navy, representatives of the National Research Council, the Rockefeller Institute, and the large pharmaceutical and biological companies. Once again, there was no argument. The need and the opportunity were again too patent.

Before the night was over fifteen thousand dollars had been allotted to start the work. The Red Cross had been invited to participate. Research, procedures, and forms of co-operation had all been laid out, in outline at least.

On June 13 the project started work.

During that summer, with the aid of twenty-five thousand dollars given by the Red Cross and with the co-operation of nine of the largest hospitals in New

York, the actual collection of blood began. Soon the donors were coming in at a rate of thirteen hundred every week. Soon over eighteen thousand donors were listed and typed and tested and giving their blood.

They were, mostly, ordinary people: hospital nurses, stenographers, clerks, housewives—the sort of people who wanted to do something every time they read the papers—but who, until then, had practically nothing that they could do. They came, with their knitting bags and their newspapers. They sat in waiting rooms and corridors. They bared their arms and watched the red fluid course through the needles and tubes into the bottles. And they went away asking when they might come again, when they might once more give their blood to save people they had never seen.

They didn't know it, those people, but while they were helping Englishmen, they were laying the groundwork for the life-saving techniques that, sooner or later, would save their own sons.

Nearly twelve million cubic centimeters of blood were collected. Over four hundred thousand dollars worth of plasma was produced. Yet not one of these donors took a penny. No one offered money. No one asked for it.

In the hospital laboratories volunteers worked after hours. Nurses stretched their working days to ten, fourteen, and eighteen hours. Doctors turned from days of operations to add nights of blood-letting and plasma-processing to their schedules. Again, not one asked a penny.

Out of it all came five thousand liters of plasma before the turn of the year, before the British caught up with their own work and were able to send word that their own production of plasma had reached a point where further shipments were no longer needed.

Out of it came something else, too. Something which, today, is more important. For doctors the country over learned new methods of collecting blood en masse, new ways of treating it, of separating plasma, freezing it, drying it, and storing it against the day when our soldiers would send out a new call.

That day, as every schoolchild now knows, was December 7, 1941. The Japs came over the hills and made for the airports as if they'd done it fifty times before. Surprise wrote the score that day. It wrote the casualty lists as well. It was because someone slept at the switch that over sixty per cent of all injuries at Pearl Harbor were burns, "flash burns" that covered and seared a man from head to foot.

Burns, of course, are not uncommon in naval warfare. But these burns were far more extensive because the gun crews had no chance to prepare for battle-station duty as they would have had if at sea. All the men had rushed on deck lightly clad and many wore only shorts.

As the Jap incendiary bullets caused one explosion

after another, the "flash" seared the skin of these un-dressed men. It left those who, by chance, were clothed almost unharmed.

A more cruel, more thorough test of plasma's use-fulness could not have been devised. For here was shock at its very worst.

Any burn is a severe injury, no matter how small, but the severity of burns increases geometrically with the size of the burn. The doctors at Pearl Harbor might have thrown up their hands as they saw case after case come off the launches and into the hospital bays with burns that even five years ago would have proved fatal.

But they had a "secret weapon" of their own and their faces did not show the worry that marked the brows of the sailors who carried in their wounded comrades. The doctors' secret had arrived six weeks before, the by-product of John Scudder's New York "plasma factory," seven hundred and fifty flasks of precious plasma powder.

It wouldn't be enough. That they knew after the first hour. However, it would tide them over until the local transfusion services got under way. For the doc-tors of Hawaii had organized donor services "just in case" and they also had a small hoard of whole blood stored away in the refrigerators at Tripler General Hospital. Even as the lines of ambulances wound into

Honolulu, the lines of volunteer donors also began to form at the hospital gates.

When, on the next day, the Mayor of Honolulu decreed that traffic fines would be paid in blood donations, he was merely expressing the awareness of all the population to the fact that blood had become as important a weapon as bullets.

The doctors and nurses at Tripler and the other Hawaiian hospitals found themselves on a seemingly endless round of duty.

First, a morphine injection, using the wonderful new syrettes—single-dose plastic packages that carried their own, sterilized, hypodermic needles. These saved a minute here, two minutes there—and hour upon hour of shock-accelerating pain in the aggregate.

Then a blood sample from each patient and a quick check against the color slides under the glass. Most of these men showed a high concentration of red blood cells, indicating a corresponding loss of precious plasma proteins and fluids.

Next a quick reference to a chart, first used by the British doctor, D. A. K. Black, who had met the same problem in bomb-pocked London. It was a simple chart, but a mighty handy one to have around when too little plasma meant death for the patient and too much meant that none might be left for some later victim.

It worked like this. The blood smear was compared

for redness against a set of standard slides. The redder and more opaque the smear, the greater the concentration of red cells in the blood stream. Then the chart showed, for every degree of concentration, just how much plasma was left in the blood stream. Simple subtraction from the norm told you how much had seeped away and had to be replaced.

The whole measuring procedure took less time, in trained hands, than it now takes to tell. A good technician could call out the exact quantity of plasma required by any case within two minutes.

With the plasma call a new device came into play, another ace the doctors had up their sleeves. For at Pearl Harbor the Army's new Standard Dry Plasma Package was first used under war conditions. It consisted of two bottles, each locked in an air-tight, sealed tin can. One contained the dry yellow powder that had started as a pint of human blood in some New York hospital almost a year before. The other contained three hundred ccs. of sterile, distilled water. Both bottles, in their tin cans, together with all the necessary needles and rubber tubing, were sealed in a waterproof fiber box.

In short, all possible protection is provided for the most precious package a soldier can carry. Yet it may be opened and ready for work in exactly four seconds. Pull a string that hangs an inch or so from the outer box and you've opened it. Pull another cord and the tight-fitting cans and all accessories come out of the box as a unit. Pull a metal tab and the cans are opened.

Again, a few seconds more or less might not seem to be important. But remember the backlog of nearly three thousand military casualties, plus thousands of civil raid victims, that confronted the doctors at Hawaii. Seconds add up, not only to hours but to lives as well.

Three out of every four in that great backlog needed transfusion. Somehow the small plasma bank was stretched. Somehow the doctors managed to get blood to every last case.

There was the seven-year-old boy from Honolulu who wasn't brought into the hospital until fourteen hours after his leg, hip, and side had been horribly burned. The poor tike was so thoroughly dehydrated his eyes seemed to be sinking into his head. So near death was he that a salt solution was injected even before a plasma dose, just to get some liquid into his blood stream. Then came plasma, a full pint. Then another pint. Then whole blood—and more blood. And drop by drop they pumped life back into the kid.

At first, just enough life to make it worth the bandages to dress his burns. Then, bit by bit they brought him back. By December 15, the child was straining at the leash. By Christmas, the hospital had a new mascot, who scampered through the wards bringing

Christmas cigarettes from the tree on the balcony to the bedridden patients.

There was the young pilot who was carried into an army hospital within the first hour of the raid. He had scrambled from his bed with the first detonations, racing across the field only to find his plane a mass of twisted, burning wreckage. Then, grounded, he turned to helping the wounded out of one of the burning hangars. A delayed-action bomb gave way on his last trip and he never found out whether there were any more men in the building. Instead he looked down to find the inside of his right hand and forearm torn to shreds. "That wasn't a blood stream," someone later said, "that was a cloud-burst."

Yet the pilot had consciousness enough to remember his training. With his left hand he put a tourniquet on the injured arm before he collapsed. When they brought him in he was a typical traumatic shock victim, drifting quietly into the coma that ends in death.

They gave him a prompt plasma transfusion, then followed it immediately with whole blood. And even the doctors, who had seen many miracles that morning, were amazed to watch the color come back into his ash-gray face. The blue ears and fingers turned pink again. The dry lips moistened. The breath deepened, first with a fast beat, then slower and more nearly normal. His eyes opened, and he asked for a cigarette.

Call it a miracle, if you will.

But remember one thing. It was a miracle that started six thousand miles away in some blood-donors' station in New York. It started with John Scudder who knew, way back in 1940, that doctors couldn't turn their eyes away from this war and who got nearly twenty thousand New Yorkers to help him develop his plan.

That plan has now grown into a great, nation-wide plasma bank. The twenty thousand have been joined by hundreds of thousands, will yet be joined by millions.

That's the real miracle.

Chapter II

"THAT SMELLY LITTLE SPANISH DOCTOR"

BY January twentieth the war was over in Catalonia. Everyone knew it; even the people knew it. And the Fifth Column managed to tell it to those who were slow at getting the idea.

Franco had broken through. Sitjes was only fifteen miles to the south and Franco's men sat there. Martorell was only ten miles toward the west and Franco's men sat there. At Manresa, thirty miles to the northwest, Franco's Germans held the town. The Falangist tongues grew bold as they whispered, "The gap is closing; flee, flee to France while there is still time."

And so the defeat that was already all but certain was hastened towards its consummation. The flood of refugees started for the north, blocking the roads to military movement, choking off what little in the way of supplies might have trickled through the French cordon.

On the twenty-second the official evacuation began. Children and prisoners marched off in groups. The ambulatory wounded walked in straggling lines, inventing weird new hobbles to eat up the dust-caked miles.

They needed whatever head-start they could get, for by the next night the flood was on for fair. Half a million bewildered people, soldiers and civilians, were on a march towards a goal that was no goal at all, towards the sealed, air-tight border of divided France.

On the twenty-sixth, the day that Barcelona fell, the vanguard of the refugees rolled up to Portbou and broke like the first black wave of a storm against the barriers of the border guards. Opposite Le Perthus they piled up on the roads and spread to the fields. From heights along the frontier, as far as the eye could see, the steady river of humanity pushed up to the thin dividing line between a land lost to Fascism and—so it still seemed—a haven.

With the neat precision of bureaucrats the French began sorting saints from sinners. If you were a deserter, you might get through under International Law as a "soldier." As the crowds grew to swarms they began to pass the children and some of the women. But still they turned back wounded soldiers and air-raid civilian casualties in a senseless series of vacillations.

Finally someone with more military sense than a border guard pounded a table and demanded action. Behind the civilians was the Republican Army. If they couldn't get through there would be a battle at

the border—perhaps an international incident! Even
Franco would rather have it over without another
fight.

Only then—and even then not without delays and
a stickling for ceremonial details—were the gates let
down at Portbou, at La Junquera, and at Puigcerdá.
At one point they poured through at the rate of four
thousand an hour, every hour from dawn right through
the night. More than a hundred and fifty thousand
civilians! More than a hundred and fifty thousand
soldiers—if you could still call these tattered, foot-
weary veterans, who barely dragged their guns out of
Franco's reach before dropping them, soldiers.

Among this ragged host were thousands of wounded,
including more than two thousand who by all the rules
of military medicine should never have been able to
leave their beds in Barcelona's hospitals. These last
were sorted out (even a blind man could have performed the tasks for the casts they bore emitted a horrible, all-pervasive odor) and rushed to special isolation hospitals, hurriedly set up by La Sanité Militaire
Française.

The French doctors were prepared for casualties.
But this? Nothing like this had ever been read of in a
textbook. Nothing like this had ever been seen, in all
their experience from 1914 to 1918! Had they fought
four years in vain, that these stupid Spanish doctors
should not yet know how to treat a compound fracture,

with constant irrigations, dressings, and antiseptics?

So ran the agitated conferences of the French military surgeons, stirred out of comfortable routines. And then, striking the group collectively, came a horrible, whispering thought:

"Gas gangrene!"

But of course. The smell. That horrible stench. The weak drawn faces of these poor men. But of course, gas gangrene. Did not they, with all their care, with all their antiseptics, have thousands of cases of gas gangrene in '16 and '17? What filthy, hideous gangrenes must be hidden under those stinking casts!

"Gentlemen," said each to the others, "gentlemen, amputations of urgency are in order."

And so they started to operate, cutting right and left. There was no time to pause. No time to think. Operate. Amputate. Save the lives if not the limbs.

Several hours and several score of amputations went by before they began to realize that something was wrong and that it wasn't the plaster casts. They began to look at the wounds under these casts and to find clean, pink, granulated tissue growing smartly.

Of eight hundred cases they examined, only one bore out their fear of gangrene.

Be it said to the credit of these Frenchmen that they admitted their mistake. They wrote it up, in fact, and reported it to their medical societies—not quite as a mistake, it is true, but as a medical miracle. In February one rushed to read a paper before the Société de Chirurgie de Toulouse. In May, another paper was printed in the journal of the Lyons Société de Chirurgie. Later Dr. M. Arnaud attested to the facts before that high court of all French surgeons, the Académie de Chirurgie in Paris.

But none of them—as far as their printed words show —really understood what they had seen. Some even suggested that perhaps there were no germs of gas gangrene in Catalonia. A handy thought, that, except that there was gangrene in Barcelona and throughout all Spain.

And still they had another excuse. Those casts had smelled so badly. The wounded had seemed so ill; their mouths so dry, their skin so drawn. Here the French savants were quite correct. And why not? The wounded had arrived after days and weeks under the psychological and physical conditions of an army in full defeat, the conditions which, traditionally, have led to the highest military mortality rates.

What they didn't quite realize was that by all their rules these men should never have been able to walk at all.

Yet walk they did, on the very casts the doctors condemned. And they arrived at the French hospitals not merely alive but in better condition than any Frenchman with a similar wound had any hope of attaining, though he lay in the finest hospital in Paris. Like it or not, understand it or not, the French military doctors had to admit that there was something more than an odor to those casts.

Thus in defeat and in exodus—it seemed at that time —did history place its seal of approval upon the method and the work of Dr. José Trueta.

Like many of the medical proponents of revolutionary ideas, Trueta does not show up well to the casual reader of his papers. He consistently manages to get into fights with people. He's constantly explaining why this one was wrong and that one mistaken. He has an explanation ready for every objection that older surgeons raise. A most disturbing, not to say obnoxious, young man. But with that same curious, all-redeeming habit of being dead-right that characterized Pasteur and Koch and Lister and Walter Reed and many another great man of medicine.

When the civil war started in Spain, Trueta was thirty-eight, rather on the youngish side to be the Chief Surgeon of the General Hospital of Catalonia, the largest hospital in Barcelona and one of the largest in all Spain. But he had already had quite a career in medicine. For ten years he had been chief surgeon of one of those large mutual benefit societies which served as the Catalonian equivalents of our accident and health insurance companies.

Trueta's society specialized in the prevention and treatment of industrial accidents. So the young doctor was not unacquainted with the problems of treating compound fractures, in peace as in war among the most perplexing of surgery's dilemmas.

As he watched other surgeons and delved into the medical literature on the subject, almost all of what Trueta found pleased him not at all. For whatever the methods the surgeons used, better than half their compound fracture cases either died or lost their fractured limbs. The seat of all their troubles lay of course in the nature of the wound, a nature suggested by the very name, *compound* fracture. Where bones were broken but the skin left whole, as in a simple fracture, no one had much trouble. If you were an unskillful surgeon, you set the bones badly and they healed out of plumb. If you were good or your patient lucky, you set them just so and in a few weeks your patient was up on his feet with a new limb almost, though never quite, as good as new.

But compound fractures were different. For not only were the bones broken, flesh and skin were torn as well, and you found yourself with the problem of inducing healing in a raw, gaping wound that seemed to provide a nesting place for every sort of infection.

No wonder then that most of the earlier surgeons used the most drastic methods in dealing with these cases. For without drastic treatment they knew them to be almost hopeless. In civil and in military practice the standard treatment called for amputation and prayer. The former removed the site of the infection. The latter was sometimes observed to be efficacious in preventing a reappearance of infection at the new wound.

Then came Lister, the great preacher of antisepsis, who applied the discoveries of Pasteur to surgery. He it was who forced the doctors of Glasgow—and later, of all the world—to abandon the dirty morning coats that were their operating uniforms and seals of office. He made them wash and sterilize. Most of all, he taught them to use antiseptics, to kill infections with chemicals, to burn bugs with acids and alkalis.

One of Lister's earliest cases, in fact, was a compound fracture. A lad was brought to him from the local fair, a lad whose arm had been horribly mangled in some machinery. They had had a fair time of it getting the boy out of the mess. He had lost much blood and the wound was already swelling. But Lister saved the boy by the simple—so it seems today—expedient of cleaning the wound and keeping it clean with his germ killer, carbolic acid.

From then on, until the present day, Listerism governed the thinking of all but the smallest fraction of medical men. The value of antisepsis was so thoroughly proved that research and experimentation tended to channelize along that line.

Carbolic acid was a strong bug killer. But it proved too strong. It not only killed the germs, it killed the tissues as well. Trueta knew how the search continued after that. He knew how many new antiseptics had been developed. And he also knew that while some were harder on the germs and easier on the living flesh, none of them really worked on compound fractures.

True, the death rate had dropped. From ninety per cent in military practice to seventy, sixty, and even forty during the last phase of the first World War. True, fewer amputations were performed. True, all this was better than before Lister's time. But it just wasn't good enough. When you started to treat a compound fracture you wanted something more than a fighting chance. At any rate, Trueta wanted more than that. And after a while he came across another man who hadn't been satisfied with a fifty-fifty chance, another medical heretic, the American, Winnett Orr.

Orr had served as a military surgeon with the American army in France in 1917 and 1918. He had wanted to specialize in bone diseases and so he had been reasonably happy when they assigned him to compound-fracture cases. Just about as happy as any sensitive surgeon could be with a death rate hovering between forty and sixty per cent. Which means that Orr had been happy to work and unhappy enough to work hard and to get some new ideas.

Then the war ended and Orr found himself with a problem on his hands unique in medical history. Thousands of wounded were to be evacuated to the States, across three thousand miles of pitching ocean. And Winnett Orr had the job of bringing back the fracture cases. The Thomas splints and other devices, which did well enough in holding the fractured bones in place in the Savenay Hospital, would never do if the ships ran into a nor'wester on the homeward voyage. Something else was needed, though Orr had no definite idea of what that something was to be. Plaster casts were in order. That much was clear. But what kind of casts?

Orr finally solved the problem by a half measure. Where the fracture wound seemed to be healing— where nice, new granular tissue could be seen—he applied closed casts, covering the entire limb with plaster, wound and all. But where the affected area had not yet reached the clean, healing stage, Orr invented a strange series of braces, combining cuffs of plaster above and below the wound with metal side bars. These allowed him to inspect and dress the wounds daily.

Up to this point, Winnett Orr was quite innocent of the crime of medical heresy. He was merely applying differing devices to differing wounds in order to secure a desired end, as nearly complete immobilization as possible during a rough sea voyage. But when he got his cargo of cripples back to the States and began to remove their casts, things didn't work out according to the rules.

The closed casts, which violated every rule because they didn't permit of drainage and dressing and antiseptic irrigations—these casts covered rapidly healing wounds. And the patients who bore them had had no pain on the voyage home. Some, in fact, had violated orders and hopped out of bed every time the orderlies' backs were turned.

The boys with the open casts didn't fare so well, despite the constant care they had received. Their progress was slow, even when good. And some just didn't progress at all.

Luckily for Orr, his use of both types of casts gave him something approaching a scientific control. He had performed a clinical experiment almost without knowing it, certainly without quite intending to do so.

Strangely enough, the same fact which Orr now observed had been noted before. As far back as the Napoleonic wars, surgeons had occasionally immobilized a wound for transport only to find that—miraculously—it healed when the rule books said it should have stayed unhealed or even gotten worse. But these earlier surgeons had written off these strange cases as freaks. Certainly no one before Orr had followed the facts straight out onto the limb of a theory.

Winnett Orr, however, just couldn't forget his mass test of closed plaster casts. He wrote a paper on the strange case, suggesting that immobilization of the wound was more important than keeping it antiseptic.

He said that the body walled off infection if both the bones and the soft tissue were immobilized. And having localized the bugs and poisons, the body fought them to a standstill, if only you let nature take its course.

And then he went back to private practice and continued to experiment with closed plaster casts. Now he put them on civil-life fractures, immediately after setting the bones and removing the dead and dying tissue around the wound. But his patients and his fellow doctors objected because the casts began to smell after a day or two. And after a week or two they no longer smelled. They stank.

Yet every time he opened a cast to find out what had gone wrong and caused the smell, he found a clean, rapidly healing wound underneath the odorous exudate. And his patients felt better. Their appetites grew, they had no pain, no swelling. They sat up. They walked. And most important of all, they recovered—more often and more completely than anyone's fracture cases had ever recovered before.

But that smell! How could anything be good that smelled so bad? That smell didn't contribute to Orr's popularity with his fellow physicians nor to the popularity of his methods. Most of them preferred to stick to the cleaner, neater, non-smelly methods of irrigation and open treatment. Which was all right, as long as no one compared results.

Then Winnett Orr applied his cast treatment to oste-omyelitis cases as well. And here he won a larger measure of acceptance, although he had to fight for every inch of it. By the late 1930's there was quite a respectable minority of surgeons who would, occasionally, apply his methods, when they thought the case just right.

And one of these was José Trueta.

Trueta not only applied Orr's methods. He seems to have been one of the very few who understood just why they worked. At any rate, when the generals revolted in Spain and most of the military surgeons went with them, Trueta had something more than a theory to go on. He had already used the closed plaster technique on more than a hundred industrial accident cases of compound fracture.

The war, however, quickly brought out another advantage of the Trueta-Orr method. In civil life the patient could usually reach some sort of operating table and some sort of surgeon within a few hours of injury. Almost invariably he made it before the "golden period" of six hours was up—the limit beyond which infection really gets going.

But in battle the problem is quite different—different enough to give a preponderant advantage to the Trueta method over any other. Let's see what makes the difference.

Jorge Gonzalez stops a bomb splinter, away up in

the front lines. His comrades rush him back to the battalion aid station. They get him there, in fact, within two hours and in good condition—if anyone with a compound fracture of the thigh can be spoken of as being in *good* condition.

There the surgeon, whom we must suppose to be a non-Tureta-Orr surgeon, takes one look at the wound and knows that he cannot possibly do more than give it a preliminary treatment. For if he sets the broken bone—in an open splint apparatus—Jorge Gonzalez is going to have to occupy a bed at the clearing station for the next two or three or four weeks. And clearing stations just can't be used for permanent occupancy. First of all, there are sure to be new patients needing the bed just as badly as Jorge Gonzalez. Secondly, the whole station may have to pack up and retreat or advance, depending upon how effective Jorge's comrades up at the front line prove to be.

So Jorge's doctor gives Gonzalez a dose of morphine, an anti-tetanus injection, and a dressing and sends him down the line in the first available ambulance. Any time from three to thirty hours later, depending on many factors affecting the best of armies, Jorge may arrive at the base hospital, much the worse for wear.

His wound, by now, is almost certainly infected. Very thoroughly infected, if the law of averages hasn't given him an unusual break. His morphine has long since worn off and he has twitched and tossed on his long ambulance journey. At the very best, he may pull through after long extra months in the hospital. But more than likely his infection will have progressed so far that he must lose the entire limb. Gangrene may have set in.

But now suppose Jorge comes up against a doctor who uses the new methods. (Incidentally, Jorge's or Johnny's chance of drawing the other kind is growing rapidly smaller.) Jorge is put under an anaesthetic and the doctor cuts away all the injured tissue. The doctor then opens up all the possible avenues of infection and packs them with clean gauze, sterile gauze that will insure drainage towards the outside of the wound. Then, while Jorge is still under the ether, he puts a firm, hard, plaster cast over the entire wounded limb. Jorge awakes, free from pain and able, as often as not, to *walk* back towards the base!

There, in short, you have the final, argument-ending fact that won the day for Trueta in Spain. Trueta was not a military surgeon. His hospital was a base hospital as far as the military were concerned. But it was a receiving hospital for air-raid casualties and these invariably included the worst types of fracture cases.

Trueta found himself performing, unwillingly, another one of those controlled clinical experiments such as Winnett Orr had performed on the hospital ships. His air-raid victims went into plaster before they left his operating tables. The military casualties—at first—

came in as fracture cases traditionally arrived, in dressings and splints.

It didn't take many weeks, nor many hundreds of
casualties, before Trueta had sufficient evidence to
prove his case. Then, happily, he didn't have too much
of a fight of it. For the military surgeons of the Spanish Republican Army were of a different breed. The
regular army doctors, most of them, had gone over to
Franco at the start. They had been replaced by young
Spanish civil doctors and by a growing corps of volunteers from abroad—men like D'Harcourt, Folch,
Bethune, Bofill, and Barsky. Both groups were men of
an inquiring disposition. Almost without exception,
they brought new viewpoints to military surgery. And
not the least of these was the idea that they really
wanted to save lives and limbs.

These men believed fervently in Democracy and
hated Fascism with so violent a hate that they crossed
borders and even oceans to fight, in their own way,
against Hitler and Mussolini and Franco. Their way
was the doctor's way, and that meant doing everything, using every means, to save the lives and the
bodies of the young men who were doing the actual
fighting. You didn't have to break such men away
from tradition. Their only tradition was the question,
"Will it work?" If you answered that question, fully
and beyond doubt, they were with you.

Soon every front-line doctor in Spain was asking for

leave to go to Barcelona. And when they got there, their eyes bulged like those of green students watching the miracle of their first operation. For Trueta's hospital was full of miracles. One of them popped up at the reception desk one day in January, 1938, when a group of doctors were brought in from the northern end of the front.

"Hello, Doctor," he said, picking out one of the visitors, "still climbing after your boys?"

"Yes—but how do you know me?" answered the surgeon. "I've never been in Barcelona before—"

The youngster laughed, shifted his weight on his cast, and held out his identification tag. "This is my first trip to Barcelona, too," he smiled. "Don't tell me you've forgotten José Montero,[1] your own mess sergeant?"

The bewildered visitor turned to Trueta and the chief surgeon shook his head in confirmation. "But his gangrene? That mess sergeant was gangrenous when we sent him down the line. I remember it well. We only reached him after fifteen hours—a whole night on the mountain. We were sure he hadn't survived. And here he is stomping around like a general on his peg-leg—"

"Peg-leg be damned," exclaimed the youth, glorying

[1] His name is not José Montero. Nor are the correct names of other individuals, who may still be in Franco Spain, used here. All other details are, however, taken from eye-witnesses or accurately documented sources.

now in the wide-eyed attention of the entire ring of doctors. "Did you ever see a peg-leg that could wiggle its toes?"

And there, in the ornate marble hall of the hospital, the soldier reached down, lifted his heavy cast, swung the stiff leg onto the reception desk, and wiggled his out-peeking toes for all the world to see.

When the laughter died down, Trueta dug out the record of the case:

José Montero, aged 23, wounded by a shell fragment in the upper third of the right leg. First-aid treatment given at regimental clearing station. Patient transferred—after long delay—to a casualty clearing station. After dressing of the wound, transferred to Barcelona, where he arrived twenty-four hours after first-aid treatment. Open fracture with extensive crushing of the right tibia. Considerable damage to soft tissues. Gangrenous patches present on skin. General condition poor. Leg very painful. Signs of severe general infection. Operation carried out at once. All tissue of doubtful viability excised. Cellular spaces, containing stinking sero-pus opened up. Enough fragments of tibia saved to constitute a bone of normal length notwithstanding great loss of substance. Wound left wide open and packed with gauze. 12,000 units of anti-gangrene serum injected in the groin. Plaster cast applied from foot to middle of thigh. Temperature remained high for two days. Began to fall on the third day, reaching normal on the seventh. Cast removed twelve days later because of intolerable stench. New cast applied and maintained thereafter until the occurrence of complete union.

"That's the end of the record, gentlemen," Trueta finished. "Today we remove José's second cast."

But Trueta was mistaken on that last detail. For that day was January 19, 1938, the day of the great "practice" air raid on Barcelona. For the next seventy-two hours, Trueta and his fellow surgeons held the strangest clinic history had yet seen. For through that reception room trooped over two thousand civilian victims of Franco's German-manned bombers.

The front-line surgeons, accustomed to the sight of wounds, confessed later that they had never witnessed anything like the scenes of those three days. The bombers came over from the sea and the first flight had been sighted some minutes before they reached the harbor. In the hospital, signal lights flashed and Trueta was called hurriedly away. An orderly led the visiting surgeons in a body to the gallery of the operating theater. And almost before they were seated, the first casualty was brought in.

Trueta explained the routines, even as he operated. He told how at first they had used an elaborate system of first-aid stations, modeled after the army routines worked out in the first World War. "But since most casualties produced by aerial bombs in an only partially defended city like Barcelona were severe, we were quickly forced to change our organization. Delay at the first-aid posts, in the beginning, had pushed the amputation rate and the death rate up. After a time the posts were abolished and the wounded brought directly to the hospitals. From then on the organization worked more smoothly and our rates, for both death and amputation, fell."

As he spoke, teams were collecting casualties in the streets and from the debris of fallen buildings. Out in the receiving rooms, orderlies were wielding big shears, cutting away all clothing from the wounded. This was essential to permit of speedy sorting of the most urgent cases from among the flood that filled the rooms and overflowed into the corridors.

Then the first case was brought in, a man of about forty. The upper third of the right humerus, the bone of the upper arm, was crushed and pulverized. An area as large as a soup plate, along the upper arm and the back of the shoulder, was torn and lacerated almost beyond recognition. To make matters worse, the man's thighbone was likewise fractured and much of the thigh muscles torn to shreds.

Luckily he had been reached quickly, this little Catalonian baker. Somehow the shattered remnants of his great stone oven had formed a sort of bridge, as they fell, arching to give him partial protection. Between the moment of bombing and the operation only half an hour had elapsed. Even so, the visitors gasped as Trueta and his troupe of assistants began to work.

"This was no case for a surgeon," one said later. "I

cursed Trueta for a show-off while I sat there, for the man was torn to ribbons. Yet, as we watched, we saw the miracle performed. The dying man was pulled right through the gates of death."

Even as the anaesthetist administered the first whiff of ether, Trueta began cutting away the injured tissue along the patient's arm and back. Deep into the wound went the scalpel and as he made incisions, Trueta calmly explained, "A wound like this, though heavily contused, will not provide a suitable field for the growth of the grangrene bacillus—or of other anerobes —if we carefully and thoroughly cut away all dead and dying tissue.

"Next, we align the fragments of bone. We save as many of the bone splinters as possible. But we take no chances. If fragments are denuded of their surrounding membrane, out they must go. We cannot hope to save them and we may lose the patient by trying unwisely.

"Now," he continued, "with our wound thoroughly cleaned and débrided, we suture it up here where we will cause no tension. But here, in the lower part, where damage is greatest, we just pack the wound with gauze and leave it open. Now we're ready for our plaster."

Working with the speed gained through long teamwork, the group around the operating table quickly and firmly wound their plaster-soaked lengths of flan-

nel over what was left of the arm, locking the fragments firmly in position, giving the tissues that support which would insure rest and prevent tension and
movement.

Then they turned to the leg. The edges of the thigh
wound were cut back and damaged muscle cut away,
as before. An assistant applied traction to the foot, the
bones were quickly set in place, and again on went the
plaster.

It all took exactly thirty-seven minutes and then
they turned to the next case.

Late the next day, as Trueta took his tired visitors
through the wards, they came across the little baker
again. He was smiling, free from pain and able to turn
with his unhurt arm and grasp Trueta's hand. A few
spots of blood were beginning to stain the surface of
the cast, back of the shoulder and down the arm. The
chart at the foot of the bed showed a temperature of
101 degrees.

Some of the doctors were worried. Didn't the temperature indicate an infection under the cast? How
could Trueta be sure that nothing was wrong? Wouldn't
a window, a hole in the cast, let them see that nothing
untoward happened beneath the blood-soaked plaster?

Trueta smiled. He had been waiting for these questions; the same questions doctors always asked—of
Orr in America as well as of Trueta. "Let's take the

questions one by one," he began, "let's consider the temperature.

"In patients thus treated a real battle against infection is taking place at the site of the fracture. Our plaster has sealed it off from the rest of the body by immobilizing the flesh as well as the bone. But the battle must be fought. Every patient's temperature chart will show a rise for several days following the application of a plaster. Not only immediately following the operation, but each time the plaster is renewed. The temperature sometimes exceeds 102 degrees and may go as high as 104, but even if the fever lasts two or three days, there is no cause for alarm, for without surgical intervention, a fall in the temperature is the rule and, within four or five days, the patient will be without fever and in good condition.

"Now, if this man had no rise in temperature, then I'd worry—then I might even cut off the plaster. But as it is, the thing to do is to avoid premature removal of the cast, for his temperature is but a symptom of the intensity of the struggle going on in the wound. Making a window or, even worse, removing the cast, would actually exacerbate the local infective process.

"I've seen many cases where—usually because of the inexperience of the surgeon in charge—the cast was tampered with after application. We're so used to watching wounds, we surgeons, so used to interfering with nature, that we can't stand to see that plaster screen the wound from our gaze. So we cut a window. Just a small window. And then what happens? Come with me and I'll show you."

Leading the doctors to the end of the hall, Trueta delved into a file and brought up a set of photographs. "Here's what happens," he said, thrusting a picture before the group. "The immobilization we strove so hard to attain is at an end as soon as the window is cut. The pressure is maintained everywhere else, however, so things are actually worse than if we had no cast at all. The wound swells—swells right through your damned window and the patient's temperature and pain and rate of pulse—all these rise to indicate the spread of infection. No, my friend, there's one thing you'll have to learn if you are going to use this method, and that is to leave your casts alone.

"Of course, we do change our casts. After all, when we apply them, the wound is still discharging freely. The discharge is carrying away the products of disintegration—a process which invariably occurs however carefully the operation has been performed. As a usual consequence we get a strong odor as the discharge soaks into the cast. Especially in hot weather, it is difficult to tolerate the first cast for more than ten or fifteen days. Then we take it off—clean the already far-healed wound—and slap on another cast. The second can usually be retained for twenty or thirty days and the third indefinitely, any time from one to two months.

"Now, with our baker here, we were lucky. His cast, you notice, is becoming soaked with blood. We get that whenever we've been able to reach a case within a few hours. Then the first cast can be maintained longer, sometimes until the fracture completely unites. It is our maxim here that when the first cast is stained with blood, the prognosis is good."

The group passed on to the recovery wards, where the victims of earlier bombings were in the later stages of convalescence. One doctor asked about cases that didn't get to the hospital in time, cases that reached Trueta after others had failed with "standard" methods.

Trueta looked around the room and then called over one of the patients, a youngish man who had already discarded hospital dress for his street clothes. "Got your pictures, Juan?" he asked. Juan ran back to his bed and returned with a set of photographs of his forearm. As the surgeons examined the, by now, completely healed wound, Trueta read the case record.

The patient, aged 32, was wounded in the forearm by light bomb fragments in one of the severe bombardments of 1937. He was immediately taken to a local hospital where it was found that he had a fractured forearm with great bruising and destruction of the soft tissues. Treatments were carried on each day by antiseptic dressings until he was admitted to us on November 27th, ten days after injury. By then the wound was enormous with swelling of all the muscles. Pus suppurated the entire forearm. The upper thirds of both bones of the forearm were fractured and the borders of the wound were covered with dead tissue. The only treatment was to immediately excise the tissue and to apply a plaster cast. The general condition and the local symptoms of inflammation improved from then on. The plaster became so heavily soaked with offensive discharge that it had to be replaced within twelve days.

By then, however, substantial improvement had taken place. The muscular masses had flattened out and the raw surfaces had begun to granulate and heal at the margins of the wound. On the removal of the second plaster, after an interval of another fifteen days, marked improvement was observed, especially in the healing around the edges. Changes of plaster were continued until union was complete.

"And that is where we have Juan, now," Trueta concluded, while the surgeons pored over the photographs.

So it was, month after month at Trueta's busy hospital. So anxious were the army doctors and local practitioners in provincial towns to try Trueta's methods that some of them began to put casts on every wound, even when tissues were so torn that Trueta himself would have amputated. Finally, José Trueta had to drop his surgery for a few days and dictate a manual of instructions. First it was published in Catalonian.

Then in Spanish. All up and down the front and in every bomb-pocked little town it was read and reread by surgeons and by harassed general practitioners who had not held a surgeon's scalpel since their student days.

The plaster-cast method became the standard technique of the Republican Army. Over twenty thousand cases were treated by it. And the ratio of successes rose to phenomenal heights. The incidence of gas gangrene and other infections—which ran as high as eighty and ninety per cent in Flanders in 1916—fell in Spain so markedly that, as we have seen, some foreign surgeons began to say that Spain contained no air-borne germs.

Though all Republican Spain knew about Trueta and his stinking, miraculously effective casts, the rest of the world knew next to nothing about them. For Spain was no land of touring physicians in 1937 and 1938. If you came, and many did come, you came to work and to stay. And you worked so hard and so long, you didn't have time to write articles for the medical journals back home. But once the Spanish war was over and the surgeons became refugees and the visitors and volunteers went home, then the word began to spread. Journals of surgery, throughout the world, began to run articles on the remarkable, controversial treatment.

Winnett Orr, out in his Nebraska hospital, had his day for smiles. Trueta had vindicated him with a vengeance. And Trueta, himself, began to find a growing number of doctors seeking him out in London where he had found refuge.

But even so, Trueta's final vindication was some months off. Munich was still in the air during the spring of 1939 and many were the doctors who still thought they had time to debate on the niceties of odor.

Yet the tide of medical thought had definitely turned. Or rather, *been* turned. For unless you wanted to hang yourself by your old school tie, you couldn't ignore the facts of the Barcelona experience. And when the war started, British surgeons were more than anxious to listen to anyone who had played a part under the bombardment of Barcelona, the bombardment that all now knew was just a warm-up for the coming bombing of London. Trueta was invited to address the Royal Medical Society in November, 1939.

He was introduced by V. Zachary Cope, the presiding officer, with eulogy such as is usually heard only about a candidate for office and then only from his campaign manager. Cope called Trueta's contribution "a momentous one, bidding fair to revolutionize one of the most difficult problems facing surgery."

The Catalan doctor then sailed into his subject and for over an hour the assembled surgeons of Great Britain scribbled notes like a crew of schoolboys. Nor were they ashamed to do so, for Trueta's lecture had a background of experience, of successful experience, of which they all were well aware. When he had finished there were only a few questions and these served but to point up the immensity of the advance which the Trueta-Orr methods represented over the "standard" practice. The bacteriologist, Dr. Leonard Colebrook, pointed out that "eighty to ninety per cent of all open wounds in the first World War became infected with hemolytic streptococci and a very great percentage of all deaths were due to the same cause. What," he asked of Trueta, "was your experience with these germs?"

"They were present," Trueta answered. "All types of streptococci were found in the wounds. But they did not produce general infection or other complications because the immobilized tissues isolated them. Of 1,073 cases, we had six deaths, and none due to streptococci."

Then Dr. C. A. R. Schulenberg arose. "Dr. Trueta had mentioned the horrible smell of the casts. Had he been able to take any local measures to combat the smell?"

"Yes," Trueta replied. "For a while we used brewer's yeast—packed it in the wound—and it worked to a degree. The yeast, in fermenting, absorbed the products of disintegration of the tissues. Our trouble was in getting the yeast. There were more bombs than brewers those days in Barcelona."

And that was all. For once the assembled surgeons of England—accustomed as they were to question every new idea—trained for generations to an "enlightened skepticism"—for once they had no questions. For what questions were necessary in the light of the record of experience? And who would have the temerity to question that record after Trueta had shown his pictures, after D'Harcourt and Jolly and the venerable Hey Groves, dean of British surgery, and Surgeon Rear Admiral Gordon Gordon-Taylor and half a hundred others had testified to Trueta's methods.

No . . . this was no time to raise hair-line questions as to the niceties of method. This was November, 1939. The same Nazi who had lent his bombers to Franco was now at Britain's heel. And providentially this man whom some had called that "smelly little Spanish doctor" was now among them with a new method of treating the fractures that make up about sixty per cent of all war injuries—a method that worked with a death rate of less than one per cent.

There was only one thing to do—and the British surgeons did it to a turn. They paid to Trueta that greatest of all medical tributes; they adopted his methods, lock, stock, and barrel, plaster, stench, and all. All they added was the one thing Trueta would have added himself—the new sulfa powders dusted into the wound.

And in America, Winnett Orr was proud to find that his method had come to be called the Trueta-Orr method.

Chapter III

DOCTOR MOORHEAD'S SECRET WEAPON

THE mid-November fog lay over San Francisco like a thick white shroud. From his room, high in the Saint Francis Hotel, John Moorhead could see only the trolleys and busses of Market Street, heading down the hill toward the harbor. His eyes picked out a car as it passed beneath him and followed it until the soft white mist fudged its outlines and swallowed it whole. Of the harbor, where his boat lay, and of the Golden Gate, through which he knew he would soon pass, not even the outlines could be seen. He knew they were there; the whistles of passing tugs and ferries would not let him forget that he was on the edge of deep blue water, but for all his eyes could see there was nothing but pea soup beyond the three-block circle the fog scribed around his room.

Dr. Moorhead turned from the window and resumed his packing. He was on holiday and nothing that happened at Post Graduate Hospital back in New York could affect him for the next six weeks. His students would have to get along without him. His patients would have to trust in Dr. Lisle or Dr. Peterson. This morning he could still be reached by phone; the devilish instrument that keeps physicians awake sat on the table before him. But within six hours—no, within less than five hours now—he would be out of reach even of telephones, with nothing to do but lie in a deck chair until Diamond Head hove in sight.

The small, white-haired, slightly stoop-shouldered surgeon smiled as he looked around the room to find some last thing left out of his trunks. There on the bed was the small black bag, the badge of his trade. He opened a drawer in his steamer trunk and pushed the socks and handkerchiefs down until he had room enough to put the tell-tale satchel out of sight. Then he turned to the small wooden box that rested on the table. He scratched his head and wondered. Would it fit in the bottom drawer with the shoes? Probably not. Maybe he'd better carry it; the stevedores might slam that trunk just once too often. Yes, he'd better carry the little wooden box.

He closed the last lock, turned the lights out, rang the desk for a porter, and walked to the elevator. As he stepped out of the car into the broad lobby a bellhop came up. "Carry your radio, sir," he said. Moorhead didn't argue with him. Come to think of it, the box did look like a portable radio.

Then, as he came to the steps that led to his cab, John Moorhead paused and felt in his inner pocket.

Tickets, wallet, and beside them an envelope. He thought of the letter in that envelope, the letter post-marked Hawaii and topped with the seal of the Hono-lulu Medical Society. As he stepped into the cab, he smiled to himself. "Holiday," he thought, "yes, a bus-man's holiday."

John J. Moorhead has been practicing surgery for forty-five of his sixty-eight years. He was a lieutenant-colonel in the Medical Corps during the last war. He has the Distinguished Service Medal of the United States Army and the French Croix de Guerre. He is the author of two of the most widely used texts on trau-matic surgery. He is Consultant to the U. S. Public Health Service. He is Medical Director of the New York Transit Systems. He is Professor of Surgery at Post Graduate Hospital Medical School and consult-ing surgeon at six hospitals. In short, at sixty-eight John Moorhead is the sort of man who might well sit back and take things easy. He is also the sort who always tells himself he will but never does.

Take that Honolulu vacation, for instance. John Moorhead got off the boat on December 3, 1941. On the fourth he gave the first of three lectures on trau-matic surgery to a couple of hundred physicians, civil-ian surgeons, and Army and Navy men. On Friday night, December 5, the audience for his second lecture had grown to three hundred, virtually every surgical man in Hawaii, with a large group of general practitioners to boot. On Sunday morning, December 7, he was scheduled to give the third and last of his lectures.

The audience had assembled and Moorhead was walking to the dais. In his hand was the brass-handled wooden box that looked like a portable radio. Inside was an instrument, the like of which Hawaii had never seen. The military men especially were interested, if somewhat skeptically so, by this gadget. They had heard that Moorhead had developed a foreign-body detector that actually worked. Well, they were ready to be shown.

But they were not shown that morning. The group had barely assembled when the secretary of the Medical Society rushed down the aisle. "Ten surgeons are needed at once at Tripler General Hospital," he shouted. Then they heard the rattle of anti-aircraft fire and knew that the planes overhead were on no routine practice flight. The meeting dispersed quickly and twenty minutes later Dr. Moorhead was in an operating room starting what turned into an eleven-hour stretch.

For a few moments there was the inevitable confusion. Some of the younger men thought old Moorhead had become rattled when he carried his wooden box with him into the hospital. It seemed to them a little like grabbing a candlestick or a coffee pot when you run from a burning building. But, if they thought thus, they dropped the idea quickly. Too many other things were forced to their attention. Those who found themselves on Moorhead's team quickly discovered that, whatever it was that made the old man run with a wooden box, it wasn't a quirk of senility. Moorhead was younger than they were when it came to working at the operating table.

And so they worked, patching here, cutting there, removing scores of metal scraps and dusting ounce after ounce of sulfanilamide and sulfathiazole into the wounds. Every once in a while, usually after removing a dozen scraps of shrapnel from a man on the table, Moorhead would turn to a nurse and say, "Take that man's name. I'll see him later." Again, the now most respectful assisting surgeons could not quite understand just what was going on, but by now they were content not to wonder. Moorhead must know what he was doing.

Then at last the relief team came up, around eight-thirty that evening. The weary doctors retired to their locker room, but most of them did not have the energy to change their clothes. They lit cigarettes and fell back on the dressing benches, closing their eyes and drinking in the smoke. Then one sat up and nudged the man next to him. Together they watched Dr. Moorhead. He sat on the bench before his borrowed locker, holding the wooden box in his lap. Gaping, they watched as he opened the kit. Inside they saw something that looked like a radio—but not an ordinary radio. This must be the gadget they had heard about. Quietly the tired group massed around the older man, so quietly that, in his preoccupation, he did not seem to notice them. Then he turned his head and the blue eyes crinkled and smiled. "Never did get around to showing you gentlemen this gadget, did I? Well, we're relieved for the next six hours. Suppose we all take a cat-nap and then, about midnight, I'll show you how to find hidden gold." The box snapped shut and wordlessly the surgeons changed their clothes and went out.

By eleven-thirty that night the group was back and waiting, augmented by a score or more of men from the other surgical teams. There, in the doctors' dressing room, Moorhead took up the lecture that had been interrupted early that morning. Now he spoke to surgeons who knew what war was really like, to men to whom the "influx of surgical cases" was no longer merely a textbook phrase.

He told them of the former methods of locating bullets and bomb scraps. One way, of course, was just to probe and hope: to wound the wounded all over again while you sought for a tiny speck of dirty metal that shifted even as you looked for it. It wasn't the method of choice under any circumstances, but in the past it had often proved to be the only method you could use when you had to remove the foreign object at once in some field hospital tent or mobile operating room.

Another method was to use the X-ray, if you had an X-ray. That was the method which, theoretically, should have been used at Tripler Hospital on December 7. But how could you propose to do so when, within a few short hours, over nine hundred and sixty cases were brought before you, scores of them foreign-body cases of the worst sort. The X-ray techniques in use varied pretty much with the whim of the surgeon using them. Some men recommended taking the patient into the X-ray room, placing him on a table in the same position he would occupy on the operating table, and examining the area in which the foreign body was located, under a fluoroscopic screen. When you found the tiny scrap of metal, you pushed a syringe needle through the skin and tissues till the point of it was seen, under the screen, to be in contact with the foreign object. Then you transported the patient back to the operating theater. As one textbook put it, "Providing the hollow needle has not become displaced whilst the patient is being transported and anaestheticised, it is a simple matter to cut down alongside the needle and locate and remove the foreign body."

Simple indeed, if you have one conveniently placed fragment. But what about the men they had just finished treating, men with twenty, fifty, or a hundred fragments literally peppered into them by bomb-bursts?

Another method called for operation in the X-ray

room. Again the textbooks gave the show away. "Its only limitations," they said, "are the size of the X-ray room, its lighting and general suitability for operative work." They did not mention another limitation, the line of waiting men that would stretch, in any real emergency, from the X-ray room to Kingdom Come.

Still another method reversed the procedure. Instead of trying to operate in the dark X-ray room, the surgeon is supposed to have the X-ray equipment brought into the operating theater. If you have a handy "special operating table with a thin aluminum top," you would then be able to put your X-ray tube under the table. If you donned a special fluoroscopic screen bonnet, strapping it to the head, you would then be able to examine and locate the foreign object.

According to the text, "There are two distinct methods of using the bonnet: 1. The foreign body having been previously localized, the operator commences the operation, and when he has reached the region where the foreign body is thought to be, he has the bonnet put on his head and, after pausing a few minutes to accommodate his eyes, the X-rays are switched on. With probe or blunt dissector he then works through the tissues till contact is made with the foreign body which he then removes under the X-rays with forceps. 2. In the second method an assistant wears the bonnet and points out the position of the foreign body in relation to the surface. He continues to do so during the various stages of the operation, until the foreign body is finally reached."

As Moorhead solemnly reviewed these methods, his audience rocked with laughter at the thought of attempting to apply these seriously written instructions under conditions such as those with which they had just been battling. Then he reviewed the multi-plane X-ray method, the procedure most generally followed in civil practice. Here, two X-ray pictures were taken of the area in which the foreign body was located. By taking one picture at right angles to the other, it became possible to determine quite accurately just where and at what depth the foreign object was located. This method was thoroughly practical, if you and your patient had time enough to go through the procedure. But it involved taking two X-ray pictures, developing the films, comparing them with the actual body of the patient, and marking the patient's body to conform with the indications of the X-ray. Then, after all this preliminary procedure, you were lucky if some slight movement of the injured man failed to shift the foreign object and destroy your entire calculation.

The audience was quite ready to grant the futility of all these methods, at least under wartime operating conditions, by the time Dr. Moorhead finished describing them. Then he brought out the wooden carrying case and opened its lock. The radio-like apparatus was withdrawn and placed on a table, while the old surgeon told them how he had come to invent his device.

"You know, gentlemen, that I served with the Medical Corps in France. But unlike many another surgeon, my civil practice, since that time, has not drifted too far from wartime conditions. I've specialized in traumatic surgery and my work for the subway and utility companies of New York has brought me far more of the kind of cases that resemble war injuries than come to the average civilian surgeon. Particularly among the subway workers do you find case after case in which a man is injured by flying scraps of metal. That's why I finally got sick of these cut, probe, and hope methods.

"Then I turned to one of the City Transit Department's research engineers, a young man named Samuel Berman. Together we developed a new apparatus which works much better and much faster than anything I know of that ever was available before. I first gave this 'locator' a trial at the Reconstruction Hospital in New York. We worked on a police officer, a man who had been in the bombing at the World's Fair two years before. With our new device I was able to locate and remove several small metallic fragments from the region of the ankle, and purposely the X-ray films were not used as additional guides.

"Our apparatus is an electro-magnetic induction device functioning somewhat like the geologists' detector of buried metals. It is highly sensitive to iron, steel, brass, and copper, as well as silver and aluminum. It is less sensitive to lead but will indicate that metal's presence. Notice this wand-like finder or probe. To use the 'locator,' we pass the probe over the area being prospected. We can even sterilize it and insert it into a wound if necessary. When the probe passes near the foreign object its electro-magnetic field is disturbed and the disturbance is measured on this dial. The higher the needle climbs on the face of the dial, the nearer we know we are to our object. Thus I can stop directly above the thing I am seeking, if I watch my dial for its point of maximum rise.

"To tell how deep the object lies, we approach it from the side and follow the same procedure. Or we note the point at which the needle reaches its maximum height. Naturally, if our metal scrap or bullet is near the surface, the needle will rise higher, while if the object is deeply buried the peak of the needle's swing will occur at a lower point on the dial.

"Tomorrow, if things have quieted down enough, we will give the 'locator' a real wartime test. There's one case in particular, a machine-gun bullet lodged in the spinal canal, that I think we can save with this 'gadget.'

"But if for the time being you'll grant me that the device will work as I say it does, you must then agree that it offers marked advantages over the old-time methods. You can use it wherever you move your hospitals. It will work on ordinary house current or even on the juice you generate by portable apparatus to work your lights. If necessary, it can be made to work with batteries, for use in regions where no installed electricity is available. Yet portability is but one of its advantages. Time-saving is even more important, as you gentlemen well know after today's experience. With a locator such as this the surgeon can find his bullet or shrapnel scrap and remove it right at the operating table, under full light, without moving the patient and without waiting for X-rays to be taken and developed.

"Finally, there is the matter of saving the patient from the further shock and trauma of an unnecessary cutting and probing. For with an accurate location of the foreign object, we eliminate a very large part of the surgical work involved in excising the metal body. No needles, probes, or scalpels need be used for mere location purposes. The only cutting that may be necessary is that which leads directly to the object of our attention. Now, gentlemen, I see that it is almost time for us to go on duty. I hope we can stage our demonstration tomorrow."

The next two days saw not only the demonstration Dr. Moorhead had promised. Twenty-two separate demonstrations were staged, first by Moorhead himself and then by the chief of the surgical service and a number of his assistants. In every case the "locator" proved helpful. They started with the simpler wounds, those of the extremities where the foreign objects were obviously restricted to a small area. Then they went on to more doubtful and more difficult cases. Finally they turned to the young soldier with the bullet lodged in his spine.

The man was brought in and placed face downward on the operating table. Anaesthesia was given to him and the big surgical dome lights overhead sprang into brilliance. All around the working team, stood tier after tier of other surgeons, men who had managed to come off their tours of duty and men who had taken time out of their hours off to see the secret weapon at work.

The wound of entry was clear in this case, the very sort of puncture a machine-gun bullet makes, right on the lower spine. Every indication showed that the missile had entered the spinal canal and lodged there. But just where within that long tubular structure no one could tell. The bullet had taken an oblique course in entering. Once it pierced the flesh and hit the bone it undoubtedly took some twisting, curving path that might have brought it to a stop at any point within quite a few inches of its point of entry. After it stopped, it may have wandered further, as the man was moved from the field where he was hit, first to a stretcher, then an ambulance, then through the hospital halls to operating room and wards.

Moorhead picked up the pencil-like metal wand with its long extension cord leading back to his instrument and dials. He carefully adjusted his rheostats and controls, then turned to the nurse who waited with a bottle of sterilizing fluid. The wand was dipped, sterilized, then inserted into the wound. All eyes froze on the needle.

At first it stood stock-still. Then as the probe moved deeper, the needle began to rise. Moorhead shifted his gaze alternately from his patient to the wavering needle on his locator's dial, although he could probably have known just how the needle moved by the rise and fall of his audience's breathing. He shifted the probe a bit to the left. The needle fell. Then right. And further right. It rose and fell again. Then right and upward, just a fraction of an inch. The needle wavered and then swung clear across the dial. The audience breathed outward as one man. Noting exactly the angle and depth of his probe, Moorhead removed the wand and replaced it with a pair of surgical forceps. A moment later he stood erect, the forceps held upright and a shiny, lopsided slug of metal gleamed and glistened between the prongs. Another surgeon stepped up and dressed the wound while the entire group followed Moorhead into the next room to examine the locator more closely.

There was little time then for congratulations or applause. In a few minutes the group dispersed. Moorhead and his team returned to their routine of operating on the wounded. But a few weeks later, just after Christmas, a group of doctors accompanied John Moorhead to the ship that would take him back to San Francisco. With a deliberate attempt at the offhand manner, the secretary of the Honolulu Medical Society took his friend aside. "John," he said, "the boys thought it would be nice if I could make a trade with you. I'll give you what I've got in this package if you'll let us keep that 'locator.' I know we could buy another soon, but we sort of feel we'd like to have this one handy—just in case Tojo visits us again."

Moorhead smiled, said, "Sure," and they both went up on deck. The "All Ashore" was being called and with the package in his left hand, John Moorhead shook the hands of each of the many surgeons who had come to see him off. As the darkened ship moved out into the pitch-black harbor, he tore the wrappings off the package that had been traded for his locator. His surgeon's fingers could easily read the incised inscription on the brass plate he found in his hands. It began, "To Colonel John J. Moorhead, in appreciation. . . ."

Back in New York, Moorhead and Berman put their heads together once more. They got out their original plans and went over them. They changed one thing and another, monkeyed with this circuit and that, till all hours of the morning, night after night. When they finished, they had come up with a new "locator"—simpler, more portable, and nearly twice as sensitive as the original.

Today, in a plant somewhere in the eastern states, scores of the new Moorhead-Berman "locators" are being manufactured. As each comes off the final test line, it enters a waiting shipping case which may take it to Australia, Africa, India, China, Ireland, England, Iceland, or Russia. And soon the lives owed to Dr. Moorhead's secret weapon will mount from dozens to hundreds and thousands.

Chapter IV

UNSEATING THE FOURTH HORSEMAN

THE bombers began going eastward almost before dusk. They rose from their hidden fields like swarms of black hawks, but to the fighter escorts above them the green-brown of their top-side camouflage made them look like nothing so much as moving sections of Britain itself as they swept over the newly plowed fields of East Anglia and Kent.

Behind each flight of bombers the fighter planes rose one above and behind the other. Pilot Officer Douglas sat at the controls of the last and highest plane and sang. His gunner, Flight Sergeant Hulbertson, didn't know what song it was he heard, but by the time they were over the North Sea he was humming the tune himself, the somber, solemn tune that beat to the deep rhythm of all the motors from every side.

They reached the coast of Holland before the moon rose. A few miles further on, they saw the flash of the Flight Leader's fighter as he swooped across the moon, turning back toward England. They turned too, Douglas trimming his plane neatly after the bank, still singing. Then a shadow came across their wing and both men knew that this was it. A Messerschmitt had them on the tail. Hulbertson jumped to his turret gun, turned it rearward and waited, while the Nazi drew closer. Cool as ever, Douglas was still singing. At two hundred yards both planes let go at once. Hulbertson could hear the whoosh of the fifty-caliber bullets as they sped by. That was all right, he knew, as long as he didn't hear the sudden stopping of their sound, the stopping that tells you one of those slugs has struck home. With the moon behind them they had a chance, in spite of the Nazi's eight guns to their rear-mounted one. Not a good chance, but a chance nonetheless.

For a second that seemed an hour, Hulbertson held his fire. Then his finger closed slowly and smoothly over the trigger and his tracers told him his aim was correct. The Nazi veered off to the left and lost altitude fast. They lost him soon in the darkness, couldn't see if he ever hit the sea.

After all the noise, it was comforting to Hulbertson to hear the song coming up towards him again. The quiet by contrast now let him hear words for the first time. Or possibly Douglas was singing louder. He made out, *"But I struck one chord of music like the sound of a great Amen."* Then he turned towards Douglas and realized why the tune this time had changed. Their motor was smoking, badly. Without really breaking off the tune, Douglas continued crisply,

"Bail out, we're going to fry. Bail out now, Hulbert-son, that's an order."

He could see Douglas cut the throttle and ignition switches and then the flames shot back. The pilot's hands went to his face, instinctively. The whole top of his body was wrapped in flame. Hulbertson saw the officer's cap float by him in the blast. He grabbed Douglas and dragged him back. The cockpit door wouldn't open but he kicked it till the lock sprang. Then he grasped Douglas around the waist and jumped. He never did know how he pulled the rip-cord but, after a while, they were both floating down and he got a new grip on his chief. Before they hit the water, he could see the small green light of a speed-boat moving towards them, attracted no doubt by the flaming beacon on the sea that had been their plane. He had to thresh water only a few minutes before they were picked up, the uninjured sergeant and the burned pilot.

The stretcher-bearers who brought the wounded airman into the hospital weren't quite sure that their chiefs knew what they were doing. Not this time, any-way. For anyone could see that the man was dying. He lay there, under the blanket, and never moved; not when they jostled him going up the stairs, not when they set him down at the admitting desk, not when they tugged at his clothes to get his identification tags and papers out. Not even when they set him down on

the operating table. It wasn't up to them to say anything, but if you asked them, the poor lad would be
better out of his misery and quickly.

The nurses soon had his clothes cut away. Two of
them worked on the still wet fabric while the third sat
on a high stool making notes of everything the others
did. "Pilot Officer John C. Douglas," she wrote, "age
27; home, Edinburgh; next of kin, Mrs. Mary Douglas;
status, wife." Her busy pen went through the routine
for the thousandth time while her eyes seemed never
to light for more than a second on the paper. She
stopped when the doctor approached, then took up
her writing again as he called out, "Petrol burns, second degree, involving forehead, nose, complete right
half of face, dorsum of right hand, forearm midway to
elbow."

"This lad will need a plasma transfusion, Miss Herbert," he continued. "Get him ready while I dress."

When the doctor returned, in his great white coat,
not ten minutes later, the head nurse had already given
her patient a morphine injection. His arm was bare
and swabbed. The plasma bottle hung on its wire
rack over the operating table. The needle pierced the
vein and the liquid began to leave the bottle. Miss
Herbert's hand, on the airman's wrist, tingled as she
felt his pulse strengthen, quicken, and rise towards
normal. Johnny Douglas moved, opened his eyes and
slowly focused on the doctor's half-masked face.

"Sorry," he said, "so sorry. . . ." Then the morphine took effect and he closed his eyes again.

They moved him into another room. The anaesthetist filled a hypodermic with potenthal sodium and shot a few drops into his veins. Douglas relaxed and drifted off into a quiet sleep. The anaesthetist fixed his eyes on Dr. Ross and watched for the flicker that, now and again, said, "Give the patient another drop."

Gently, the doctor took a swab of cotton, soaked it in ether soap and scrubbed the wounded man's face. Slowly, yet without a wasted motion, he went over every inch of the burned area. Then again, this time with a salt solution, removing each loose bit of singed skin. The nurse handed him an atomizer filled with a brilliant purple fluid. The raw, exposed skin began to glow as the dye stained it. Then, with the hot-air blast of a small hair-dryer, Dr. Ross worked slowly over the purple areas, which dried to a dark, smooth, filmy sheen.

The physician next took up a soft artist's paint brush. Like a painter working a background in, he daubed the purple areas over again, this time with silver nitrate. They were all breathing a little easier now; the youngster wouldn't die, not yet at any rate. But the air was tense with their fears of a few moments before, until the doctor broke the spell. "Remember the Nazi we had here last week, Miss Herbert?" he asked, without stopping his painting. "The orderly in the prisoner's ward told me he nearly died when he saw the black stains of this stuff on his arm. He thought we were marking him so that he couldn't escape."

"His kind would think that," Miss Herbert answered and went back to her pulse-counting. The doctor finished with the second fluid and took up another spray, tannic acid this time, applied mainly to the arms. When he was done with it all, the lad was taken to a bed and placed under a shock cradle, a wire contraption covered by a blanket and heated by two large electric bulbs. They gave him another small injection of morphine and left a nurse to watch him.

He came to the next morning and watched the doctor while the whole painting process was repeated. His temperature stood at one hundred degrees for all that day and half the next. He had no pain and almost no swelling. By the third day they could no longer keep him tied down. His only complaint was that "the damned black stuff" kept him from opening his eyes all the way. But in another day the coagulum began to peel. It came away from the eyelids first. By the eighth day, large areas of healthy pink skin were coming to view. In another week, Pilot Officer Douglas was completely healed with no trace of scarring or contracture.

Burns and war have marched hand in hand ever since Babylonians first shot flaming arrows over city walls. But in today's war, burns are more numerous, deeper, and more extensive than ever before. One does not have to look far to find the reason for this change. Mechanization and particularly the motorization of fighting make for those "accidents" that produce severe burn injuries, often of types not commonly found in civil life.

The pilot is particularly susceptible to flames attacking the face. He throws his hands up to shield his eyes and wakes, if he wakes at all, to find face and hands seared crisp. The seaman and especially the gunners and passers of naval ships are often enough the victims of flash burns, speedy explosive flashbacks that sear off any uncovered skin in half a fleeting second. Sixty per cent of all the wounded at Pearl Harbor were in this group, augmented in severity that day because but few of the men were dressed when the early-morning attack was made. Merchant sailors have to add the risks of floating on burning oil to the already considered risks of torpedoing or aerial bombing. Civilians and soldiers alike must meet the menace of the fire bomb, a weapon known to the ancients but multiplied ten thousand times in its destructive power by the development of aerial bomb-sowing and of chemicals which burn at intense heats.

Yet though the incidence of burns has climbed in this war beyond any previous level, the terror of burns today is measurably lessened; for, in the last twenty years, more has been learned about the nature of fire's effects on man and about how to fight these effects than was discovered in all the ages before. So much, in fact, has been learned that not all of it has yet been digested. Doctors who once had no good way of treating a severe burn, today find themselves with a confusing choice between competing methods, each of which is better by far than anything that we have had before. Where once the doctor could do little if anything, today his problem is that of selecting the particular method of burn treatment which, in each separate type of case, will produce the best results.

From 1914 to 1918, the world was given a mild foretaste of fire as a wounding agent. Yet the last war produced little if anything new in burn therapy. Most burns were treated as they had been treated for a hundred years before. Bicarbonate-of-soda dressings or salt solutions were used to cleanse the wound and soothe the pain. Morphine was used for severe cases. Where facilities permitted, as they seldom did at the front, patients were immersed in salt-water baths. Oils of one sort or another were smeared on the burned areas.

Practically none of these were new methods. In fact, only two or three relatively minor innovations in burn treatment came out of the first World War. One was the use of picric acid as a dressing material. Gauze was soaked in a weak solution of this acid, which served, to a limited degree, to coagulate the tissues, forming a membrane over the burn that tended to isolate it from the air. This eased the pain and encouraged healing; but picric acid dressings were very difficult to remove, so difficult in fact that they usually carried with them a large part of the newly healed tissue and thus left the victim as badly off, if not worse off, than before.

Another development, popular particularly among the French, was the use of paraffins of a type that melted at low temperature. These were applied either with a brush or a spraying apparatus and served to seal off the burned areas for a time at least. They were easily removed, but they cracked under movement and thus lost most of their sealing quality. The method was somewhat painful, for the paraffin had to be applied hot. Daily dressings, with accompanying daily pain and renewed opportunity for infection, served further to limit the usefulness of this method.

Towards the end of the war, a variation of the Carrel-Dakin solution, Dichloramin-T, was sometimes used, either in conjunction with paraffin or as a separate spray. Here the effect sought was antiseptic, but the method has long since fallen into disuse.

The real trouble was that no one really knew just what happened to the body when it was burned. Theories there were aplenty. But for every theory there was another that contradicted it, in whole or in part.

Most theories were, in fact, merely that and nothing more; the ideas of men who came across a few burn cases in the course of years of practice and who drew conclusions based upon their limited observations. For in civil practice burns were not particularly attractive to the older, established physicians, the men who headed large hospitals or controlled the investigations of great research institutions. People would, of course, get themselves burned. Between five and seven thousand persons died every year, in the United States alone, from burns. But almost nine-tenths of all burns were household accidents, the sort that were naturally treated, if treated by physicians at all, by the ambulance interne. Even industrial burns seldom got the attention of the big men. Usually the plant doctor or some local general practitioner was called in, as with any other accident case, to do the best he could by the use of traditional first-aid methods.

Thus when some great conflagration or the advent of war finally brought the problem face to face with the medical profession as a whole, even the older doctors found themselves forced to fall back on the experience of their own interne days. It is perhaps for this reason that most of the important work that has occurred in the last twenty years has been done by young men; men who became interested in burns because they saw far more of them than their elders did.

The one great exception to this rule was Frank Pell

Underhill, who first began to study the nature of burns and of their effect on the human system in the early 'twenties when he was already past forty-six and had to his credit many lasting achievements in other fields of chemistry and medicine. At first glance his interest in the subject came about as the result of an accident, the great theater fire which occurred in New Haven in 1923. Underhill and a group of his associates participated in the treatment of twenty-one of the victims of this fire and utilized the opportunity afforded by the number and severity of the cases to make extensive studies. A closer examination of Underhill's early history, however, shows that this was merely a milepost along a path he had long been traveling.

Frank Underhill graduated from Yale University in 1900. He remained at Yale first as a graduate student, later as instructor and then successively as Professor of Pathological Chemistry, Experimental Medicine, and Pharmacology and Toxicology. He might have remained until his death within the Yale cloister but for the first World War, which brought him into the Chemical Warfare Service as a lieutenant colonel and took him to France as the United States delegate on the Inter-Allied Gas Warfare Conference. Thus, during the war and for some years thereafter, Professor Underhill concerned himself with the effects of war gases on the human system and the methods of treatment best suited to counteract or minimize these effects. Much of what we know today on this subject we owe to the original researches, conducted at Yale and elsewhere, by Underhill.

With the occurrence of the great influenza epidemic of 1918, Frank Underhill was struck with one outstanding similarity between the effects of this disease and those of war gases. Both gave rise to swelling within the lung tissues and both brought about high concentrations of the red cells of the blood. Calling upon his knowledge of the treatment of war-gas injuries, he was able to suggest similar methods of treating these effects of influenza. And so, when he again came upon similar symptoms among his fire-victim patients, Underhill was prepared as was no ordinary physician to attack the problem from a new and more basic angle.

Although scattered work along some of these lines had been done by others in earlier decades, Underhill and his associates first clearly demonstrated the fact that burns caused a loss of fluid into the burned area and thence out of the body itself, and that this fluid loss resulted in concentration of the blood. On the basis of Underhill's work and that of others inspired by the signposts he nailed up for them, the treatment of burns was tied closely to the general treatment of shock of all kinds. Doctors began to try to compensate for the lost fluids in order to prevent or alleviate the condition of shock which such fluid loss induced.

Deaths from shock, which once caused two-thirds of all burn deaths, began to drop off a bit.

In 1930, shortly before his death, Underhill carried his work much further on an experimental basis. On controlled burns, inflicted on anaesthetized laboratory animals, he was able to prove that the fluid lost into the swelling burned area was essentially the same as blood plasma. Measurements showed this to rise as high as seventy per cent of the total blood volume. Given this direct indication, others were able to carry the problem on to its logical solution and to develop the techniques of plasma extraction, preservation and transfusion which, today, are a mainstay of all anti-shock treatment.

Thus, under the inspiration of a Yale professor, hundreds of workers have gradually uncovered the secrets of the nature of burns. Many of the crude theories and old wives' tales have been exploded. Today, burns of a severity requiring hospital treatment, and many less severe, are recognized as wounds having profound effects on many of the body functions and on many organs located far from the region reached by the fire. A whole system of *general* treatment, to counteract these *general* effects, has been developed. The doctor pays quite as much attention to the patient's general condition as he does to the burned areas. Blood counts are a routine. Plasma injections are given in all severe cases and whenever the blood count indicates that blood concentration is occurring. The effect of new understanding and the treatment arising therefrom cannot be measured accurately, simply because burn deaths have been cut by new local treatments as well as by the general treatments. But few indeed are the cases with any hope of life which die from burn shock today.

While Underhill was testing his theories by the blood counts of the New Haven theater victims, a young man just past his first interneship was making a discovery that has since revolutionized all local treatment of burns. Edward Clark Davidson was the brilliant son of a doctor father, the sort of lad who is president of his class and, at the same time, a star center on the basketball team, editor of his high school literary paper, and vice president of the athletic association. No one was surprised when he romped through Harvard in three years nor when he graduated with honors from Johns Hopkins Medical School. When he served a year as interne at Johns Hopkins Hospital he seemed to have started on the proper path towards a fine practice or perhaps a Johns Hopkins professorship.

But then Ed Davidson did something his friends thought out of character. In June, 1921, he turned up at the then quite new and not yet renowned Henry Ford Hospital in Detroit, for an additional year of interning. Most young doctors would have looked upon

Ford's as just a branch of the motor plant, a sort of glorified first-aid clinic by which the wizard of the Model T hoped to combine the kudos of the philanthropist with the economies of treating his own industrial accidents. But young Davidson knew what he was doing. Ever since the days when he had sat in his father's Pittsburgh office and watched the men from the mills brought in with hot-metal burns, he had had a hankering to do something about these cases that no one else seemed to care about. At Ford's he knew he would get such cases, for fast-drying lacquers had not yet been introduced into the auto industry and paint-room explosions were a commonplace in all the Detroit factories.

So, at twenty-seven, the young interne began to chase after burn cases. Soon every such case that entered the hospital was turned over to Davidson both because no one else particularly wanted them and because he was showing quite a knack for treating them successfully.

At the time—and even today—a large number of burn theories centered about the idea that the burn itself produced toxins which poisoned organs remote from the burned areas and even the body as a whole, bringing on severe illness and frequently death. Davidson subscribed to the particular branch of this general theory which saw the burn toxins as proteins; parts of the body fluids in some way converted by the burning into body poisons. Instead of trying to treat these poisons when they manifested themselves by their poisoning action in the blood stream, at the liver, in the intestines, or elsewhere in the body, young Davidson sought for a method of attacking the proteins right at the burn site. He could find plenty of proteins there, for the body fluids that keep a burn weeping and the edema fluids that cause swelling around and under burns, are high in protein content. Davidson figured that if he could find some chemical that would unite with these proteins when they were still in the burned area, he could keep them from turning back into the body to act as poisons. After one or two tries with other chemicals, he hit upon tannic acid, and, sure enough, he was able to precipitate his proteins by pouring a weak solution of tannic acid over the burned areas. The precipitate took the form of a leathery coating on the skin or skinless flesh, a coating which the doctors called an "eschar."

Under this eschar, the burns rapidly healed. Somehow, very few of the patients developed the general toxemia which so many had formerly succumbed to. The tannic-acid treatment, however, did more than Davidson had first intended for it. It covered over the raw nerve ends and thus eased pain as soon as it was applied. It seemed to speed up the healing process. It served, to a high degree, to ward off the infectious bacteria which contaminated so many burns, converting seemingly rapid recoveries into fast-sinking relapses. In short, it worked.

It worked so well, in fact, that within a year the method was being widely adopted everywhere. Improvements began to come from one source or another, all over the world. Someone tried spraying on the tannic-acid solution instead of using wet compresses as Davidson at first did. Someone else worked out a jelly that could be applied in first-aid work. Everywhere, doctors began to record an amazing drop in the mortality of burn cases. In New York, Doctors Bancroft and Rogers adopted tannic acid and cut mortality from forty per cent to twenty. Doctor Beekman, treating burns among railway workers, cut mortality from 37.8 per cent to less than 15 per cent. Dr. James Mason, in Philadelphia, lowered the death rate from 28.5 per cent to 13.3. From Europe the same sort of reports began to flow in; William Wilson in Edinburgh had been losing nearly forty per cent of his patients. But tannic-acid treatment cut his rate to 11.1 per cent. In Vienna the rate was sliced from 16.3 to 7.7. Finally, from London came the report of Dr. P. H. Mitchiner with a death rate quartered to an all-time low of 2.4 per cent.

No wonder, then, that the conservative *Surgery, Gynecology and Obstetrics* was moved recently to state, "Perhaps not in this century has one surgeon accomplished so much in the saving of life, the lessening of suffering and the saving of patients' time and money, as has E. C. Davidson by his work first published in 1925." Ed Davidson, himself, lived long enough to see his method win world-wide acceptance and to carry his clinical and investigative studies much further. When he died, in 1933, of that doctors' malady, heart disease, he had converted burn therapy, from something tossed at the youngest men because others wouldn't be troubled, into a thoroughly scientific branch of medical research. He did not live long enough to see his own methods largely—but by no means entirely—superseded by newer discoveries. But those who knew him, through his work or through his writings, know that far from resenting the changes that have overthrown some of his theories, Davidson would have welcomed them as the logical growth of his chosen branch of medical science.

Just about the time of Davidson's death, another youngish man, Robert E. Aldrich, began to attack another aspect of the sickness brought on by burns. Where Davidson had sought to fight burn poisons, which he could not quite prove were actually present, Aldrich proposed to go after the bacteria which he could very definitely prove infected a vast majority of severe burns.

It is a curious commentary on the workings of the human mind to note that hundreds of papers have been written by hundreds of doctors who speculated about burn toxins, which none of them, not even Davidson, have ever been able to isolate, while no serious study of the ever-present bacteria in burns was made until young Aldrich got on to the problem. Somehow, it was easier to erect theories about the unknown, easier to speculate about a new toxin different from everybody else's toxin. Since 1923, more than twenty different toxic agents have been seriously proposed as the guilty parties, a pretty good indication of the confusion of thought on the subject. But getting down to the dirty, tedious work of following each patient from the time he entered the hospital, of taking culture after culture of burn fluid, blister fluid, and blood, of tracing the growth of bacteria and their effect on the patient—that was the sort of hard, unrewarding work which once again fell to the lot of a youngster.

Bob Aldrich, however, was no mere laboratory hack. He not only was able to prove that bacteria infected most burns within twelve hours and caused many of the later complications which led to burn deaths or prolonged convalescence; he was also able to find a way of fighting off the bacteria before they really got going. He first used an aniline dye, gentian violet, which coagulated the burn surface much as did tannic acid. But it also acted as an antiseptic, particularly against the hemolytic streptococci which found in the wounded tissues of burns a fine, lush breeding ground.

Aldrich's gentian-violet treatment had a number of

advantages over tannic acid, at least for certain types of burns. It could be applied by spraying without any preliminary cleaning of the wounded areas. It went to work earlier and spared the patient much of the pain of cleaning a dirty burn. As recovery began, the dye formed a softer and much more flexible eschar than did tannic acid. One of the main advantages was the fact that it seemed to save the tiny, almost invisible islands of skin that even a severe burn leaves. These are usually destroyed under tannic acid and thus gentian violet tends to give a faster regrowth of skin and faster general recovery.

Unlike Davidson's discovery, Aldrich's was not universally and immediately accepted. It has stirred up an almost endless controversy and doctors who now specialize in burn treatment grow violent at medical meetings as to the relative advantages and disadvantages of dyes and other antiseptics versus tannic acid. Yet, with the years, Aldrich's method has won a steadily growing number of proponents. In 1937, after several years of work, Bob Aldrich brought forth a new antiseptic-coagulant which has become known as triple dye. By combining three aniline dyes, the original gentian violet, brilliant green, and acriflavine, Aldrich secured an antiseptic that was effective against most, if not all, of the bacteria which might conceivably attack a burn.

Triple dye has another advantage, which proves of

particular importance in the deeper and more extensive burns characteristic of this war. Under a tannic-
acid crust any infection that may occur is masked and
cannot be seen until it begins to affect the patient's
general condition. But the thin translucent crust of
triple dye changes color and becomes moist and soft
over any contaminated area. Thus, while the infection
is still localized to a small area, the attending physician can locate it quickly and lift up and cut away the
triple-dye coat at that point. Cleaning away the infection, he then resprays the area and the patient continues on his route of recovery undisturbed.

The tannic acid versus triple dye controversy has
been further complicated by the fact that a modifica-
tion of either method, combining the original coagu-
lant with silver nitrate, has its own very active groups
of supporters. Silver nitrate has the effect of sealing
off the fluids coming out of a burn much faster than
does tannic acid. Used in conjunction with tannic acid
it forms a thinner coagulum and thus goes part of the
way towards meeting the objections of the proponents
of triple dye. When used in conjunction with gentian
violet, the silver nitrate likewise forms a good seal
against fluids, while letting the underlying dye act
against infections. Thus, after almost endless and very
violent arguments, the compromise between the two
types of treatment, the heavy tan of tannic acid and

the light coating of antiseptic triple dye, seems to be coming into general favor.

To add to the seeming general confusion, there are still two other methods which are widely used, not to mention an almost infinite number of variations. The first of these is the recently developed sulfadiazine spray devised by the American, Dr. K. I. Pickrell. This is sprayed on every hour during the first day, every two hours on the second day, every three hours the third day, and every four hours the fourth day. Military surgeons are somewhat chary of it, if for no other reason than because it requires so elaborate and time-consuming a routine, hardly the sort of thing that can be carried out while tending a constant stream of casualties. But the results gained by this new method are quite spectacular and, fully aware of the growing importance of the sulfa drugs as a basic antibacterial treatment, doctors are doing a lot of experimenting with the Pickrell sprays and may possibly work out some more effective and speedier method of using the sulfa drugs. In England, sulfanilamide pastes and jellies are being used, with reports indicating good results.

The second of the newer methods is, once again, the development of a young man, Surgeon Lieutenant-Commander John Bunyan of the Royal British Navy. Bunyan's approach to the problems of treating burns represents a revival of a method that long antedates the development of tanning, the use of continuous warm baths. These had been largely abandoned since Davidson's day because they required special equipment and special attention such as would not ordinarily be available at the scene of an accident or even in the average hospital and would certainly not be practicable under war conditions. John Bunyan, however, figured that if he couldn't bring the patient to the bathtub, he might be able to bring the tub—in modified form—to the patient. With the co-operation of William Stannard, a British silk manufacturer, Bunyan devised a whole series of fabric envelopes, made of waterproof, air-tight, plastic-treated silk and so designed that they could block off any section of the body, from a hand to the entire trunk. Each envelope is equipped with exit and entrance spouts through which salt solutions may be pumped.

In Britain, where the Bunyan envelope has received wide application, it has been found to have great advantages. It is easily and quickly applied and can even be put on at the first-aid station or in the tight quarters of the smallest war vessels. The treatment is painless and the envelope allows and, in fact, encourages full and free movement of the limbs. This last quality is particularly important in preventing loss of movement and skin contractures on burns of the hands and feet. Skin grows over the burned areas rapidly and the growth can be watched and studied through the envelope's transparent walls, without removing the protective coverings. Finally, for the very difficult cases, such as burns combined with compound fractures—a type of wound often suffered by airmen—the Bunyan method offers the possibility of treating both wounds as one. In combination with the sulfa drugs, applied locally under the envelope, the method provides a high degree of protection against infection.

As you read of the wide variety of methods recently developed for treating burns and of the differing opinions of the doctors who advocate each method, you may conclude that such confusion spells a pretty raw deal for the wounded. The confusion, however, is more apparent than real. In the first place, all of these methods are infinitely superior to anything, literally anything, available during the last war. This has been proved time and again, in civil life and in the war to date. Each has its place, being preferable for certain regions of the body or under certain circumstances. Tannic acid or tannic-plus-silver-nitrate is still the most widely used, particularly for large, severe burns of the limbs or trunk of the body. Gentian violet, gentian-plus-silver-nitrate, and triple dye are used for face and hands and genitalia and for the creases under joints such as arm pits and knees. Since they tend to save skin remnants for regrowth and since their thin coating leaves less scarring and fewer contractures of the scarred tissue, they are ideal for fingers, hands, and any other portion of the body where skin contraction would injure circulation or cause ugly distortions of appearance after healing is complete. The sulfa sprays and ointments are likewise suited principally for face, hands, and feet.

The important fact is that the terror has been taken out of burns by a whole series of new methods arising from our knowledge of what burns actually do to the injured. Today the military surgeon, the flight surgeon, and the naval doctor all know how to fight pain with quick injections of morphine, how to fight shock with plasma transfusions, how to fight infection with sulfa drugs and antiseptic dyes, how to seal off the burned areas against loss of fluids from within the body and against contamination from outside. The young men, Davidson, Aldrich, Bunyan, Pickrell, and a host of others, have, piece by piece, step by step, solved the problem their elders were once too busy to bother with.

Chapter V

NEW FACES FOR NEW MEN

THE battle is over; the wounded have been treated. Speed, science, and skill have combined to save many lives. Hearts that once would have stopped still beat: limbs that once would have been amputated rest, grow strong, and walk again. Fevers drop. Bandages are removed. The wounded see themselves for the first time.

This is the moment every soldier fears. In the tense, demanding struggle of battle he may be among the bravest. But lying in a bed, day upon day, he cannot help but wonder. "They've saved my life. I grow stronger. Soon I will leave this hospital; soon I will go home. But will it be 'me,' the old me of strong hands and a wide smile, or will it be some strange, distorted ghost of a man with a face from which, in all kindness, people must turn away?"

Every doctor and every nurse who served in a convalescent ward during the last war has seen these thoughts. For these are thoughts that can be seen. They creep like dark clouds over the bandaged faces of the wounded. They shine from the eyes of those whose eyes are all that can be seen between the swathes of bandage. These were the thoughts to which the surgeons of 1918 could offer no answer except to patch and to hope and perhaps to patch again and hope again.

Today things are different. True, the art of surgical repair is still a limited one. Lost limbs cannot yet be restored; lost sight cannot yet be replaced. But much that never could have been done in any war before can now be undertaken with fair certainty of success. And much that was once attempted in the face of failure rates of seventy per cent and upward is now performed as a routine with failures the relatively rare exception.

Plastic surgery, once looked down upon by most doctors as half fraud, half rich man's luxury, has progressed since the last war mainly in its ability to guarantee its results. The surgeon who attempted even the simplest of skin grafts in 1918 could never assure himself that the graft would "take." The transposed skin might live and grow, and then again it might blister, become infected, separate, and die. Even when, under the hands of such skillful artisans as Sir Harold Gillies, the grafts "took" successfully, the cosmetic effects of the repairs were all too often nothing to boast about. When old-time plastic surgeons wrote about their work, they adopted the manner of moralists, and, from necessity, preached that beauty isn't all, that restoring function was an end in itself.

They were right, of course. The new skin that closed an open wound was something for which to be thankful, even though it might prove somewhat hard to look at. But somehow, as the years passed and their "functionally restored" patients found themselves isolated from love, from work, and from the world itself by the ugliness of their scars, men grew to hate their saviors, these doctors who had restored their features but failed to restore their countenances. Doctors began to wonder whether much was really gained if a plastic restoration ended by driving the patient into a psychiatric ward.

But step by step, through the twenties and thirties, the plastic surgeons have learned how to control their effects. Today their specialty, which was once all "art," has become largely a matter of applied science. Predictable results can be achieved with a high measure of certainty if prescribed steps are followed. This difference in the ability to secure and to insure results is exemplified in the work of Dr. Earl Calvin Padgett, whose fame and whose instruments have spread from his native Kansas City to every corner of the globe. Padgett began to specialize in skin grafting only in the late twenties. He therefore had all the experience of such earlier workers as Blair, Waldron, Pickerill, and

Gillies at his command and, for a time, he was satisfied to walk in their footsteps.

The transplantation of skin, as a serious surgical procedure, had started in France around 1870 among physicians confronted with the wounded of the Franco-Prussian War. It soon spread to Germany and England and by the first decade of the present century there was quite a number of surgeons in many countries doing work in this field. The earliest experimenters had based their hopes of success on their observation that skin had the power of regeneration or regrowth to a higher degree than most tissues. They had noticed how skin spreads outward from the edges of a wound, attempting to cover the area which had been laid bare. They had seen skin, abraded to a fraction of its full depth, growing back to normal thickness and health. They remembered how, in wounds where large flaps of skin had been left without underlying flesh, these flaps had not always died despite the partial loss of their blood supply. Instead, some such flaps had taken root again when pressed back into place.

"If skin can grow again at its original site," they reasoned, "why can we not transplant it to another portion of the body and have it take root there?" They tried it and it worked—not by any means always nor even in a majority of cases, but often enough to prove that transplantations were possible and that failures indicated faulty techniques which might be modified and improved with time.

The ability to transplant skin may seem, at first glance, somewhat like borrowing from Peter to pay Paul. True, the new site is improved in appearance and perhaps in function. But what about the donor site, the place from which the skin contribution has been taken?

Here the doctors split into two schools of thought. Some reasoned that the important thing was to improve appearance or function. Their patients would be better off with a scar on the leg, they said, than with one on the neck or face. So they cut away the skin from the thigh and permitted a scar to form there, using the contributed skin to repair some more visible portion of the body. Others reasoned differently. Instead of cutting all the skin away from the donor site, they cut a thin sliver off the top of the skin for transplantation. Thus the donor site was left with enough skin tissue to allow it to regenerate its top surface.

Both methods had their advantages and their defects. Nor was Padgett the only one aware of them. With the Thiersch or "Split" graft, a razor-like knife was used to cut the top third or top quarter of the skin away. Relatively large areas of grafting material could be taken by this method and, even in years past, a "take" at the new site occurred at least three quarters of the time under the hands of a skillful surgeon. But these thin grafts had three principal defects, all of them important in dealing with certain types of wounds. First, their appearance was none too good. Second, protection of the underlying tissues—the prime function of skin—might prove insufficient and the graft itself might be too thin to withstand hard use in later life. Third and most important was the factor of contracture. For a thin graft contracted like rubber, often as much as sixty per cent, drawing the repaired tissues into a mockery of normal, human flesh.

The full-thickness grafts had the advantage of giving a more normal appearance after a perfect "take." They contracted little if at all. But, on the other hand, the percentage of such grafts which "took" at the new site was low. Over new tissue forming to repair a wound (so-called granulating tissue) the possibility of a good take was too slight to make the use of a thick graft of much practical value. Even with a clean, denuded surface a partial "take" was often experienced with loss of sections of the graft due to blistering.

Both the thin and the full-thickness grafts had their zones of ideal use, special types of repairs for which they are still used as the method of choice. But in between lay a wide majority of cases for which neither type of graft was perfectly suited. As Padgett and other surgeons worked on the problem during the twenties, they began to feel that some intermediate thickness of skin might combine the advantage of the two extremes and minimize the disadvantages.

The problem, however, was easier to state than to solve. For skin cutting was an operation performed by hand with the aid of a sharp knife and a sharper eye. It was hard enough for the surgeon to cut skin thick or thin. It was next to impossible for him to cut it accurately to some predetermined intermediate thickness. For here they were dealing with hundredths of an inch. The thin or Thiersch graft must be less than one one-hundredth of an inch in thickness. Cutting by hand, the surgeon could judge his depth only by observing the transparency of the peeling skin. The full-thickness graft was easier to cut, since you were dealing with a less fragile membrane and separating it from a different type of underlying tissue.

In 1929 the first major improvement in the technique of graft cutting came when Vilray Blair introduced the intermediate or "split" graft, using a specially designed apparatus to stretch the skin for more accurate cutting. With this apparatus a very skillful surgeon could control the depth of his knife and cut grafts a little thicker and a bit more accurately than before. This represented an improvement in technique and, insofar as it was an advance toward the middle ground between thin and full-thickness grafts, it provided better results. But it called for the highest skill on the part of the surgeon, the sort of skill which only a few men could hope to acquire. Padgett, for instance, confesses that even with the aid of the Blair apparatus, he was never able to cut a graft without considerable variation as to both thickness and size.

From his observations on hundreds of cases, Padgett was led to the conclusion that a graft representing three-quarters of the thickness of normal skin would be ideal for most operations. It would leave enough skin at the donor site to permit of quick regeneration and regrowth. Yet the graft would be thick enough to provide adequate protection and to minimize contraction. At the same time, such a three-quarter-thickness graft would match the surrounding skin as to texture and color.

To cut such a section with accuracy, however, it would be necessary to develop a new cutting instrument—something that would be free from the fallability of the human hand and eye. In 1930 Padgett turned to a fellow professor at the University of Kansas for aid. Professor Hood was a mechanical engineer. The team of Padgett and Hood, so it then seemed, combined all the requisite skills for the speedy development of a skin-parer par excellence.

But cutting skin presents somewhat formidable problems. For seven years the two men, both busy with the pursuit of their teaching and their professions, spent their free time inventing, constructing, and discarding skin-slicing gadgets. But try as they would to put some guard on the knife blade to keep it cutting at an even depth, their tools never seemed to work properly. The same blade that cut a given thickness on one trial produced a sliver half as thick again on the next trial.

Finally they had an idea, the sort of idea you think of at four o'clock on a sleepless night. Up to then they had been trying to hold the blade at a fixed distance from the top of the skin. They had failed because there was no way of making sure that the top of the skin would stay put. But suppose the top of the skin could be attached to something fixed, something hard. Then if you fixed your blade a set distance from that hard surface, it would be cutting the skin to a constant even thickness. That was in 1937 and it was not until the next year that they finally had a model that really worked and was ready for mass production.

The Dermatome, as they called their instrument, consists of a half-circle drum of polished metal which can be rolled against the skin. Attached to this, and parallel to its central handle, is an adjustable knife. Two calibrated screws permit the surgeon to set the knife blade at any determined number of thousandths of an inch from the surface of the drum. By painting the drum and the skin with a sticky adhesive and rolling the drum over the selected area, the knife can be made to plane off a rectangle of skin as large as the entire face of the drum, four by eight inches. This graft, unlike the most skillfully hand-cut section, is amazingly uniform in thickness.

Nor is this the only advantage of the instrument. With it, skin can be cut to an exact pattern to conform to the shape of any wound. All the surgeon has to do is to nullify the properties of the adhesive by painting the areas not to be removed with a solution of talc and ether. This prevents adherence to the drum at the selected areas and lets these rejected portions of skin pass safely under the moving blade.

With his new device Dr. Padgett could experiment with grafts of any desired thickness. He could cut thin and thick grafts better, more evenly and more quickly than anyone had ever cut them before. Moreover, he could cut far larger grafts. For instance, in the years before he invented the Dermatome, his thin grafts averaged about ninety square centimeters in area, less than two inches by two. With the Dermatome he has been able to *average* four times as large an area per operation. In many an instance he has taken the full capacity of the Dermatome, eight times his former average, at a single operation. And in a few cases he has transplanted three drumfuls at a sitting.

When Padgett chose to use his three-quarter-thickness graft to replace old-style full-thickness grafts he raised his average cut from twenty-nine square centimeters to 188 square centimeters. In one case four whole drums of skin were transposed to a single patient. Patients with extensive loss of skin, such as are common among war-wound or air-raid-burn victims, can thus be treated in a single sitting, or, at most, two sittings, whereas formerly they would have had to be subjected to a long series of painful transplantations if they could be saved at all.

The Dermatome has still other advantages. Formerly most large grafts were removed from the thighs, which were easier to cut from than other areas. When burns destroyed most of the skin of the legs and thighs, such cases often proved hopeless. But with the Dermatome, skin can be removed easily from the abdomen, chest or back. Thus the military plastic surgeon has a larger reservoir of available donor areas than he ever had before.

Since 1938 Padgett's methods and his Dermatome have been taken up throughout the world, although doctors have by no means abandoned all other methods of skin grafting. Padgett himself would not recommend so drastic a step, for each method has some advantages in certain types of cases. But the Dermatome has proved most helpful precisely where injuries of a military nature are to be dealt with, as, for instance, in and about London in reconstructing the victims of air-raid bombs and burns.

In London, too, another major innovation in plastic surgery first made its appearance. The sulfa drugs have virtually licked wound infection and infection, remember, has been even more an enemy of the plastic surgeon than of any other surgical specialist. For infections create pus. And pus literally lifts the graft away from the underlying tissues, preventing adherence or "take" and destroying the newly formed blood supply that keeps the transplanted skin alive. Failure due to suppuration or the formation of pus may be caused by any of a large group of organisms. Certain of these, in fact, appear to have a specific affinity for newly applied grafts. The worst of all, because it is the most prevalent, is the hemolytic streptococcus, the germ which according to Colonel Leonard Colebrook infected seventy to eighty per cent of all open wounds during the first World War.

There was little that could be done about this bug until the advent of the sulfa drugs. Doctors washed the areas intended for grafting with various antiseptic solutions. Often they swathed the wound in gauze bandages and kept these saturated for days with Dakin's solution or a solution of boric acid. Changes in dressings were often most painful to the patient. In particularly painful cases the victim was placed in a tub and immersed in a salt solution.

With the discovery of the sulfa drugs and the development of knowledge of their effectiveness against most bacteria, surgeons naturally tried them for skin-grafting purposes. At first there was much conflict between those who insisted that sulfa drugs would work

only when given internally by mouth, and those who,
like Colonel Colebrook, insisted that local applications were ideal for localized infections. But, as is so
often the case, the theoreticians were routed by hard,
practical facts. Wounds sprayed or dusted with sulfanilamide crystals quickly became clean and free from
infection. By the use of this method it became possible
to free an infected wound of its hemolytic streptococci
within three or four days and meanwhile the patient
suffered no pain.

One of the first doctors to follow this procedure was
John Converse, a young New Yorker who found himself in London at the beginning of the war and who
did much plastic work, during the big blitz, at the
American Hospital in Britain and at the Park Prewitt
Hospital. Converse kept records of over a hundred
cases of infected granulating wounds, records which
left no doubt as to the efficacy of the local use of sulfanilamide.

In eighty-one of Converse's cases the wounded were
infected by the hemolytic streptococcus. Twenty-one
cases resulted in failure of the graft to "take." Of these,
twelve were cases in which sulfanilamide was not
used. The rest represented infections by a strain of the
bacillus resistant to sulfanilamide. (Fortunately such
strains now succumb, for the most part, to the more
recently discovered sulfadiazine, which was not yet
available at the time of Converse's work.) Five of the

remaining sixty cases were grafted while the bacillus was still present in the wound. Even so, the sulfanilamide worked well enough to give an average "take" of seventy per cent. And in fifty-five cases, where sulfanilamide was used to free the wound of the hemolytic streptococcus before grafting, the "take" averaged ninety-three per cent. Thus, even with a drug which has since been improved, Converse was able sharply to reverse the normal expectancy of "take."

If his sole object had been to devise a process of clearing up infections prior to grafting—a process that would be less troublesome to the doctor and less painful to the patient—Converse of course succeeded. But beyond this success lay another of even greater importance. For the grafting of war wounds is often resorted to as a means of making possible, at an earlier date, secondary operations of major importance to the patient, particularly such operations as nerve suture, tendon suture, or secondary bone surgery. In such cases, skin healing may be achieved in ten days or two weeks when grafts are used, while waiting for the body to develop skin by growth from the edges of the wound may take many months. Thus the sulfa treatment is the first step in time-saving which leads to the second step, skin grafting, which in turn is essential if the limb is to be restored to its full function.

Converse and his associates first freed the wound of pus by means of dressings, baths, or mechanical irrigations. In some cases, reached early enough, they were able to use sulfanilamide immediately and thus prevent the formation of purulent exudations. Naturally, whenever this was possible, the procedure was to be preferred. But when pus had already formed, failure to remove it would prevent the sulfanilamide from taking effect. Once the wound was freed of its exudations the sulfanilamide powder was blown over the tissues. Then without waiting for the powder to take effect the skin grafting operation was performed. It had been feared, at first, that the very presence of the powder would prevent the graft from taking to the underlying tissues. But in practice it was found that the sulfa was gradually absorbed into the blood stream and far from hindering the "take," it virtually assured success.

Given his two new tools, sulfanilamide and the Dermatome, the reconstructive surgeon is now in a position to attack his work with measurable certainty of success in all except the most difficult cases. Yet this by no means describes the limits of reconstructive surgery today. The largest field for the plastic surgeon will no doubt continue to be that presented by cases of burn injury.

But the reparative surgeon must and now can restore function and appearance as well to most wounds. In many cases his work now plays an important part in fostering recovery in addition to insuring that the end result shall be of a more normal appearance. War wounds with extensive skin loss are frequently followed by marked contraction and constriction, which in turn tend to cause disturbances in the blood circulation. Thus a vicious circle is set up which can be broken only by the restoration of an adequate skin surface. The scar tissue on the healing wound will limit circulation and limited circulation will retard healing. This is particularly true in wounds of the extremities when the area of destroyed skin entirely encircles the limb. In such cases the plastic surgeon no longer waits until the regular doctors are ready to turn the patient over to him. He is called in at the very beginning because his work serves to break the vicious circle and thus permits restoration of both flesh and function.

When skin destruction is near a joint, contractures caused by healing and scar formation may badly affect the function of the limb below the joint. Thus, in many such cases in the past, contractures of scar tissue forming at the neck have bound the head to the chest or shoulder in a horrible distortion of the normal human position. With the new assurance of a successful "take," an early grafting over such a wound can assure freedom of movement and a restoration of the normal looseness of skin in this area. In many another case, similar contractions once caused inability to straighten the knee, the fingers, or the elbow. The early practitioners of skin grafting could not promise their patients that their grafts would not aggravate such situations rather than alleviate them. Today, however, Padgett's Dermatome, with its accurate determination of graft thicknesses, permits the plastic surgeon to calculate and anticipate contractions with almost exact mathematical certainty. Knowing just how much contraction is likely to occur with any given thickness of graft, he can extend the joint and fix its position in a splint so that exactly the right size of graft is utilized.

Another major type of grafting operation, using skin flaps rather than free grafts, has long been in vogue and its use in this war represents no spectacular advance except insofar as improved techniques now permit surgeons to be more daring and more ambitious in their operations and thus to achieve more extensive and satisfactory results. The skin flap or pedicle is a piece of tissue detached from its underlying support except for a small portion of one end. Through this connection it receives its blood supply while growing attached to its new site. Thus a flap may be cut from the forearm. The arm is splinted into position so that the free end of the flap may be attached to a site on the neck. The patient remains with his arm in this awkward position for a number of days, long enough for the flap to take root at the new site. Then the remaining joint to the arm is cut away and the flap end put into its place on the wound.

Modern methods of plastic surgery and particularly the use of sulfanilamide nowadays hasten the healing period and make more certain the success of the "take." The awkward position need thus be held for a much shorter time. The surgeon may also dare to utilize a larger pedicle without fear of the flap dying while awaiting the development of a full blood supply at the new site. Such flaps of flesh and skin are used principally to repair wounds where a defect of contour must be eliminated. Thus many of the ugliest wounds of warfare, the lost chins and noses which so shock the eye, can today be repaired with far greater ease than was once possible. Fewer by far will be the soldiers who survive this war with lips distorted into a perpetual grimace or with eyelids drawn into a constant squint. Fingers which have had a joint amputated may be extended with material taken from some less visible portion of the body. Bare bones on the bottoms of the feet can be given new heels by the same process.

There is still another phase of plastic surgery which has recently received much attention in Great Britain and which may yet prove to be a life-saving procedure of major importance. It finds its origin, strangely enough, in a research project which Earl Padgett initiated in 1931, a project which produced almost totally negative results.

Padgett was interested in the question of whether or not transplantation of skin from one individual to

another was a practicable procedure. If such transplantations could be performed with success, they
would open up tremendous vistas for reparative surgery. Patients too weak to withstand ordinary grafting
operations could then receive grafts from skin donors
just as they today receive blood from healthy blood
donors. The problem of what to do about the patient
who has lost so much skin that he simply cannot provide enough uninjured skin to permit of grafting would
be solved once and for all.

Padgett knew how the idea had intrigued the early
plastic experimenters. But he also knew that most of
the recorded attempts in this direction were failures.
The few alleged successes were of a most dubious nature. He therefore decided to end the controversy by
making an extended series of tests under accurately
controlled conditions.

He started with ten recorded cases for which adequate data was available. To these he added thirty-
four more cases of his own, cases in which he deliberately attempted cross-grafting. In almost every case
the first results were most encouraging. The grafts usually "took." At the end of a week, all but three of his
own cases were in good condition. By the fourteenth
day however, nine of the seemingly successful "takes"
had separated and the grafts had died. Three weeks
after operation only sixteen cases still showed a satisfactory "take." A week later this group had fallen away

to eleven and after five weeks all but four cases turned out to be failures.

These four proved most interesting. They represented the cases of two pairs of identical twins, each of whom had given a graft to the other. These grafts lasted indefinitely, until the patients were finally discharged. Padgett was not satisfied to let the project rest at that. He went back over his records and compared the blood types of each of his donors and recipients. Doing so, he found the grafts that failed immediately were those in which the blood types were antagonistic to each other; cases in which the skin donor could not have been used for blood donation purposes. Whenever the blood groups of donor and recipient were compatible, a "take" of skin transplant was almost certain. But within a few weeks the transplant, which had seemed so healthy at first, sloughed off and died.

Padgett's conclusion was that transplantation of skin from one person to another was not a practicable procedure except in the rare case of identical twins. He explained the temporary "take" in the other cases by the theory that the recipient's body took several weeks to develop a reaction to the strange skin. Until then, as long as the blood of recipient and donor was compatible, the graft actually "took" just as a self-graft would. But once the reaction set in, the body rejected the strange skin, developing some sort of "reaction serum" which caused the foreign graft to be destroyed.

For Padgett's purposes, at that time, this answer was sufficient. But in England cases have arisen where even a temporary graft would prove of great value, cases in which only a partial dressing of the burned or wounded areas could be secured at one time with the injured man's available skin. Padgett's long-forgotten research was remembered and the whole question was reconsidered. The English doctors reasoned that skin was an ideal dressing for a wound under certain circumstances. Thus, if the purpose was merely to seal off the wound, to encourage growth under the skin-dressing while waiting for the patient to grow stronger and better able to give more of his own skin; if this was the aim, cross-grafts might well be utilized. Padgett's Dermatome, which you will remember was invented long after his own experiments in cross-grafting, made possible the taking of several skin grafts from a single section of the body. All the surgeon had to do was to wait until the donor area healed, say for ten days or two weeks, and then he could tax the same area all over again.

In the British experiments the time element worked out to perfection. Consider a patient with very extensive burns of both legs and thighs, burns so extensive that not enough skin could be taken from back and abdomen at the first operation totally to repair both legs. Unless you could find enough skin, you would have to leave some areas to heal by scarring until, at a later date, the donor areas were able to give a second donation. By then the neglected ungrafted areas might have become infected. Short of this, they would certainly be delayed in their healing. The patient's general condition would resemble that of a man who had needed a graft and had not been given it.

If, on the other hand, you combined self-donated grafts with those taken from another donor, you could predict that the foreign grafts would die off after approximately three weeks. But by that time the patient's donor areas on back and stomach would have regenerated. Thus he would have had all the benefit of a skin-dressing, protecting his wounded flesh and encouraging undergrowth, while waiting for his own skin to become available in sufficient quantity.

The application of the new technique has so far been limited to a few cases. It may develop that the method has drawbacks that are not now apparent. But to date the reports are most encouraging. Men are walking about, healthy and whole, who might have died but for a skin donation that tided them past a difficult period.

Chapter VI

NO MORE TETANUS

SOME bacteria go after the human race year after year, in fair weather and foul. Since they're almost always making trouble, bacteriologists and doctors have had plenty of reason to counter-attack them. And, since they're always around, the doctors have had plenty of opportunity to study the commoner bugs and to develop their methods of fighting them.

There are other kinds of bacilli, however, that crop up here and there, that come and go in waves and cycles. These have proved harder to defeat. Fewer are the doctors who learn to know their habits. Few indeed have reason to specialize in their study. Even when the desire to defeat these bugs exists, the opportunity is something you may have to wait for—sometimes for years.

Some bugs, in particular, present a real threat to mankind at large only during wartime. Then the special conditions of war, the greater difficulties of sanitation, the crowding of masses of men into small areas, the lowering of resistance by fatigue, hard work, long hours, and hunger, all these combine to give the war bugs their opportunity.

Then usually, the doctors know too little—and learn what little they do know too late.

So, in fact, it has always been with bacillus tetani, as mean and poisonous and tricky a little enemy as Mars ever released from his bag of ill winds. For the tetanus bug doesn't attack a man unless he's down. It waits, for days or for years, for its opportunity. It waits till a man is wounded and needs every ounce of his strength to fight his wounds. Then it strikes. It crawls into the wound. It slinks through the tissues into the blood stream. It moves through the body till it strikes at the nerves. It seeks out the most vital nerve centers, in the spinal column, where it paralyzes entire regions of the body.

Worst of all, it avoids attacking the mind. It subjects its victims to the most horrible of tortures; it causes a man's own muscles to choke the breath from his body. And all the time it leaves the brain clear to suffer the terror of slow, painful, inevitable death.

Tetanus is the bug that used to kill more than ninety per cent of its victims by slow torture. But before you become too terrified at the thought of tetanus, let us put on record one all-important fact.

Tetanus has been fought to a standstill—defeated.

It began because a Frenchman once looked for a better way to fight diphtheria. Because the football players of the Naval Academy got tired of being laid up on the sidelines for days after every spike scratch earned in practice. And because a group of Navy doctors had an accident in 1937 and managed to turn a minor medical scandal into a major medical victory.

Tetanus, or lockjaw, is an acute infectious disease caused by the poison given off by the tetanus bacillus during the growth in the body tissues. The germ itself is quite common. It is found in the intestinal tracts of horses, cattle, sheep, barnyard fowl, and rats, mice, and other rodents. It is even found in the human intestines, at times—but it is harmless to man there.

It passes into the soil through the excretions of animals (and man, of course) and, once in the ground, it forms spores, becoming highly resistant to destruction. It can survive the heat of summer and wintry cold. It can even resist the chemicals which are used to kill off other barnyard germs.

As a spore, it lies and waits, against the day when it can find favorable conditions for its growth once more as a germ. It may be picked up on the feet or on soiled or sweaty clothing. But it will do no more harm than any other dirt—until it gets into a wound.

Once in a wound—the deeper and more neglected the wound the better the tetanus bug will like it— it begins to vegetate. It doesn't attack living tissues, but depends rather on the devitalized tissue resulting from a wound. If any secondary infection gets into the wound, that is raw meat for the tetanus bug, for it can then grow on the off-thrown materials created by the other germs.

It also fattens on antiseptics, the strong types that devitalize tissues. These prepare a fine bed for the tetanus bacillus, yet they find it hard to kill off the tetanus infection itself. For unlike most other germs, tetanus doesn't need an army of bugs to conduct a successful invasion. People may succumb to the assault of tetanus growths that start with amazingly few spores, so few in fact that they might escape detection even at the hands and under the microscope of the most expert bacteriologists.

The reason for its virulence is not hard to understand. Few people get tetanus, as compared with other infections. Those who do get it seldom recover. Thus there aren't scads of people walking around with acquired immunities to tetanus, as there are with a number of the more common germ diseases. Bodies which could throw off the attacks of large numbers of germs of other types, thus succumb to a few tetanus spores.

Bacillus tetani favors deep wounds to which air cannot gain access. But, in a pinch, it will take any wound. Shallow ones, with scabs covering them, it finds quite acceptable. It has been known to utilize blisters, frostbite sores, superficial burns, and even scratched insect bites as its avenues of entry into the system.

Once in the body it travels—in ways about which

there is still some dispute—to the motor horn cells which cover the nerves controlling the muscles. Here its poison, one of the most deadly and terrible known to man, causes the nerves to stimulate the muscles into violent contraction.

The first signs of tetanus usually come about a week after injury, just as the patient begins to think everything may turn out all right after all. It starts with a stiffness, or as the doctors call it, a "trismus" of the lower jaw and neck. This is soon followed by fixation and immovability of the jaw, caused by the spasm of the muscles which ordinarily facilitate chewing.

As the tetanus poison spreads, it attacks the muscles of the arms and legs and, later, of the trunk of the body. Spasms occur more frequently and are brought on by the slightest provocation. One of the most shocking of sights is to see a far-gone tetanus victim assume the arched position known as opisthotonos, with only the head and heels touching the bed. This occurs because the back muscles are far stronger than the stomach muscles. When all the muscles of the trunk go into a contractual spasm, the back muscles overpower those of the abdomen and literally lift the body off the bed.

Yet all the time the patient's mind is clear. So clear that he literally watches his own death approach as the respiratory muscles are finally attacked and breathing becomes impossible.

Death comes by asphyxia.

It comes to an untreated case, almost inevitably. But until the first World War all cases were untreated. All the doctors and nurses could do was to ease the pain with opiates. In all the wars for which records are available, prior to 1914, tetanus killed between eighty and ninety per cent of its victims.

Even during the first months of 1915, tetanus was killing ninety per cent of those it attacked. After that, with the battle lines stabilized and first-aid systems better organized, the rate was beaten down. Surgeons began to use a tetanus antitoxin as a routine for all wounded men. If they got it into the wounded fast enough, some at least were saved.

The German armies averaged a seventy-five per cent mortality among tetanus victims throughout the war, with even higher figures at the beginning and a gradual decline as the years passed. They had a relatively high incidence of tetanus cases, too—thirty-eight per ten thousand wounded.

The British fared better. They cut the incidence of tetanus from an initial rate of fifty-two per ten thousand wounded to an average of only fifteen for the entire four-year period. Only fifty per cent of the British tetanus victims died.

The Americans, because we got into the war later, when techniques of antitoxin use were more nearly perfected, fared best of all. Only two out of every ten thousand casualties (including those not of the expeditionary forces) developed tetanus. And of these, only one in nine died.

The decline from the ninety per cent death rates of the Franco-Prussian War of 1870 proved conclusively that it wasn't where you fought that counted. The soil of northern France had been fertilized by manure for centuries. Naturally it was rich in tetanus spores. Yet, given halfway decent tools, doctors could cut the rates of tetanus mortality from ninety per cent to eleven per cent, in the very same localities.

The new tools of 1915 were two in number: antitoxin and speed. The antitoxins had been developed, like many others, in the by then routine ways taught by Pasteur. But their civilian application had languished. Neither the public at large nor the doctors felt the dangers of tetanus infection important enough to warrant giving the antitoxin for every minor wound, especially because many people suffered pronounced serum sickness when inoculated with antitoxin. They hated the idea of going through a week of light fevers, sore arms, nausea, and general malaise to ward off a disease they probably didn't have in the first place. Doctors who insisted upon injecting the antitoxin were looked upon as alarmists and other doctors got the next calls.

It was not strange then that these same doctors, called into the French, German, and British armies by the war, looked upon antitoxin as something to be used sparingly. They waited, in 1915, until the symptoms of tetanus appeared. Then, when they rushed for antitoxin it was—often enough—too late for it to do much good. In fact, there are those who maintain that in the entire French army, from 1914 to 1918, there was no single case of the successful use of antitoxin *after* tetanus symptoms set in.

The army doctors learned their lessons quickly. In a few months they had the laboratories working overtime making antitoxin. They began to inject every wounded man with it, as a routine. If the wounded soldier reached them soon after his injury was incurred, he usually didn't develop tetanus. On borderline cases, the symptoms sometimes developed but the antitoxin still got to work early enough to help the body fight off the tetanus poisons.

Thus, all through the war, the tetanus rates dropped. Yet proud though the doctors might be of their World War I records, they could not help but contemplate the fact that their methods were still cumbersome and by no means foolproof. There was something inherently wrong about giving a man immunity to tetanus only *after* he was wounded, i.e., only *after* the germs had had a good chance to start their work. Too many things could go wrong that way. Too many things did in fact go wrong. The men who still died were the ever-haunting evidence of this. They were the ones who got the injections just a little too late.

The professional military men had their complaints, too. They didn't like the fact that their men knew they had to get injected with antitoxins quickly after even a small scratch. It took too many of the slightly wounded out of action. It ruined morale. Yet how could they blame their men? How could they deny a man the right to protection when even a small scratch could spell dread tetanus?

Before further research could get started, the war ended. Tetanus became again a rare infection principally affecting farmers, slaughterhouse workers, and shepherds. For such cases, the antitoxin seemed adequate. At any rate, the infection itself was so rare that few continued to worry about it.

Even at the fountain head of immunity research, the great Pasteur Institute in Paris, other problems seemed more pressing in peacetime. For instance, Georges Ramon went to work there on the problems of diphtheria immunization. For many years bacteriologists had been making antitoxins by giving a light and controlled dose of diphtheria to an animal and then taking its blood serum for processing and injection into humans. In fighting off the poisons of diphtheria, the animal developed antigens in his blood which negated the power of the diphtheria bacillus to harm him. And these antigens, transferred to the human blood stream, gave the human a high degree of immunity.

Yet there was one basic trouble with diphtheria anti-toxin. It included in its make-up not only the good antigens but also the bad diphtheria toxins. Unless it was handled just so, it might do more harm than good. Even if it didn't get out of control from careless handling, even if it didn't actually give the candidate for immunization a dose of the very disease he was trying to avoid, still it might provoke all sorts of reactions. Many people were markedly allergic to diphtheria antitoxin or, as it is more properly called, toxin-antitoxin, since it contains both poison and anti-poison.

Ramon saw in this last fact the very nub of his problem. If he could only separate the toxins from the antitoxins, every schoolchild in France, in the whole world for that matter, could be immunized. No longer would the ignorant be able to confuse an occasional accident, an occasional reaction into a general condemnation of all vaccination. A safe, foolproof anti-toxin—a detoxified antitoxin—with that perfected, compulsory vaccination could be enforced the world over. Diphtheria could be defeated once and for all.

All through the twenties Ramon and his crew were busily at work on this problem. Very successful work it proved to be. They found a way of making what they called an "anatoxin" by treating the antitoxin with formalin. Under proper controls this procedure detoxified the antitoxin, leaving it with antigenic powers unimpaired. In fact, it did much more than the old antitoxin; it provided greater and more lasting immunity. For the toxoid—as English-speaking doctors soon began to call it—conferred a lasting immunity. It stimulated the body, into which it was injected, to produce its own antitoxins. And particularly when the diphtheria bug attacked an immunized child did the toxoid go to work, producing floods of antitoxins in the blood stream that fought off the infection before it could really get under way.

Ramon had achieved what he had specifically set out to do but he did not spend much time dressing up in frock coat and opera hat to receive the medals of provincial mayors. Ramon was obsessed with the idea of multiple toxoids. He was a practical Frenchman. He knew the people hesitated to let anyone jab a needle into them and force some strange substance under their skin. Children became frightened. Adults found it too much trouble to take all kinds of injections.

Suppose you could work up some broth that would fight not just one disease, but two or three with a single injection, some super-toxoid that gave its recipients active immunity against a whole shoal of diseases? That would be something worth going after.

And that, in fact, is why Ramon went after tetanus. For tetanus really has little in common with diphtheria. One attacks mostly children. The other goes for the wounded of all ages and sexes. The symptoms and the courses of the two diseases are almost entirely dissimilar.

Yet the two diseases did have one thing in common, a thing which Ramon—as a bacteriologist—was quick to note. Both diseases produce soluble toxins. "Exo-toxins" the doctors call them, since they are thrown off by the bacilli. It was upon this element of solubility that Ramon had based his invention of formalin pre-cipitation, using the formalin to get the toxins out of the mixture of toxin-antitoxin. Presumably the same process could be applied to a tetanus-infected serum.

They tried it and again it worked. Ramon now had two toxoids and could experiment with combining them, injecting both at once. But before he did that, he had to find a place to try out his tetanus toxoid. He had to know for certain that it would do its job. But where do you turn to find tetanus victims? In all France only a few hundred people got the disease in a year. How could you tell who might be wounded or scratched—and who of those might become infected?

Ramon turned to the French Army. There he found a ready welcome, particularly from the cavalry men, who thought not only of their troops but of their be-loved horses. "Yes, they would certainly like something to protect their mounts from tetanus. It was sad to lose a well-trained horse because of a scratch earned on maneuvers. It was sad, and it was expensive. The cavalry would certainly like a tetanus toxoid for its

horses. As for the men, well, that might be troublesome. Suppose Ramon would just try his stuff on the
horses first and then, later, they would talk about the
men."

So, starting about 1926, Ramon began testing his
stuff on French cavalry horses. The French cavalry had
some sixteen thousand horses in all and, after preliminary tests, Ramon managed to get the army to
inject his toxoid into every one of them. With this test
group they would be able to prove, pretty conclusively,
whether or not his toxoid would work. For Army records showed that four out of every thousand horses
got tetanus each year. Thus if Ramon could really do
what he said he could do, they would have far fewer
than sixty-four cases of horse tetanus in the first year
of immunization.

They waited and watched. And nothing happened.
Literally nothing. Horses went through the same field
maneuvers they had always gone through since time
immemorial. They got the same broken legs, the same
scratches, the same leg wounds. They walked in the
same dirty yards, trudged through the same mud-
slogged roads, jumped the same fences and landed in
the same fertilized fields. Yet not a single horse got
tetanus. The change was not a qualified one. It was
that dream of all bacteriologists, a total victory over
disease. After that, no one quibbled about affording

Ramon the opportunity to immunize the men of the army.

Meanwhile, although Ramon had been publishing his results from 1926 onward, the rest of the world was just beginning to wake up to the import of his tetanus discovery. While diphtheria toxoid took the world by storm, it was not until 1934 that tetanus toxoid manufacture began in this country on a commercial scale. Some experimental work had been done, earlier, by a few Americans, but like Ramon, they found that they couldn't really work effectively until some large group could be induced to make a mass test with tetanus immunization.

The Navy was the first to see the opportunity and in June, 1934, an experimental project was started on the Hospital Ship *Relief* under the direction of Commander W. W. Hall of the Navy Medical Corps. Hall wanted particularly to find the ideal method of injection and the proper interval between injections. Another question that needed answering concerned the number of injections needed for successful immunization.

Hall started his experiments on a group of some fifty volunteers, using the plain formalin toxoid as developed by Ramon. But halfway through the tests there appeared a new type of toxoid, in which alum was used instead of formalin. So Hall added another question to his list and tested the new toxoid against the old. He broke his body of volunteers into groups and gave each group a different series of injections. Some got a dose at four-week intervals. Some waited six weeks between doses. Some waited eight weeks, and some even longer. Before each dose was injected, a blood sample was taken from the men and the quantity of antitoxin generated by the previous dose measured. Thus, the method which produced the best results with the least trouble—to both doctors and men—was soon discovered.

This first experiment produced a number of interesting results. For one thing, Hall became completely sold on the alum-precipitated toxoid. It proved to be a far more efficient immunizing agent than the old toxoid, giving uniformly higher blood readings. For another thing, Hall found that the longer the interval, up to eight weeks, between the first or "sensitizing" injection and the second dose, the better the results obtained. But even hurried doses, at intervals as close together as two weeks, gave a high degree of immunization.

By 1937 the first experiment had justified itself sufficiently, by its results, to lead to a larger mass test. Hall was sent to the Naval Academy where he teamed up with Captain R. Hayden, then Senior Medical Officer at Annapolis. They looked around for a group of volunteers and soon found them on the football field. These men had a special interest in Hall's experiment, for they knew, as perhaps no other group did, just how much of a nuisance the ordinary antitoxin could be.

Every time a man got a scratch on the practice field, the doctor attached to the training squad insisted, and quite rightly, on giving the injured man a dose of tetanus antitoxin. Whereupon the rest of the squad held its breath for two days to see whether the player would develop a serum sickness or an allergy. Many a man was laid up for a week and some men were kept out of important games because of such reactions. Yet the antitoxin gave only a two-week immunity and many a man had to go through the nasty process two and three times a season. Naturally they were all for anything that promised protection without these drawbacks.

So, once again, much was learned. Again, no single individual failed to develop an adequate blood level of antitoxin. By 1938 Hall and Hayden requested and received permission to make the largest mass test of all, to inoculate the entire student body of the Academy, some twenty-three hundred men.

Here was an ideal group for study. It was large enough to eliminate chance variations in individuals as a factor of importance in the resulting statistics. And it would be an easy group to control and follow up, for the men would be around for years, either at the Academy or with the fleet. They could be watched and re-examined over a long period and the incidence of tetanus among them could be compared with that of their fellow officers of earlier classes.

Hall and Hayden went into the pharmaceutical market and purchased enough toxoid to immunize their entire group. This was the largest batch of toxoid yet produced in this country and a number of biological product houses competed for the order. It went to one of the leading houses which, since it had never made tetanus toxoid before, set up special equipment to do the work. When their alum-precipitated toxoid was ready, it was sent to the laboratories of the National Institute of Health and subjected to tests prescribed by the Institute. It passed all tests with flying colors.

At the Institute they first injected guinea pigs with ten times the normal dose for humans. Since no symptoms of tetanus appeared in any of the test animals, this proved the toxoid was fully detoxified. Then one cubic centimeter of toxoid was injected into a control guinea pig weighing exactly 350 grams. Again the toxoid did exactly what it was supposed to do. The injection produced two units of antitoxin per cubic centimeter of blood serum in the test pig.

So, having taken every precaution their earlier experience led them to believe necessary, Hall and Hayden started their mass test. They lined up their twenty-three hundred middies, swabbed their arms clean, prepared their needles and began their injections.

They were just a mite disappointed with the results of their first injections. For ten men reported to sickbay. Eight had sore arms. Two had a slight fever and didn't feel any too well. And one developed a condition known as urticaria, resembling that of a man stung by wasps.

They had hoped that there would be no reactions whatsoever. Certainly nothing beyond a few slightly sore arms. The earlier tests were the basis for this hope but, still, ten reactions among twenty-three hundred men were nothing much to worry about. That would still be far, far less than if antitoxin was being used. Far less, even, than with Ramon's formalin toxoid. And none of these reactions were severe, as were those sometimes experienced with formalin toxoid.

The two doctors waited the eight weeks their routines called for before giving the men their second dose. By then, they knew, the first dose would have sensitized their bodies. The second injection would then cause the blood stream to throw up large quantities of antitoxin as a defense against the disease. For the body fails to distinguish between the toxoid, which contains no toxin, and the toxin produced by the tetanus germ itself. Provided the basic immunity has been set up by the original dose, the introduction of more toxoid will "fool" the body, as it were, and lead it to create additional defenses. It is not unusual for these additions to rise to ten or twenty times as much as is created by the first dose.

But when Hall and Hayden got started on their second round of injections they were in for a rude shock. Reactions were noted from the first. By the time they had injected eighteen hundred of their twenty-three hundred midshipmen, they had had fifty reaction cases, five times as many as in all of the first series.

Thirty-eight men had sore arms. Seven had fever and malaise. Four developed urticaria. And, finally, one man developed a frank case of shock.

Something was obviously wrong and there was nothing to do but stop the use of this batch of toxoid. Yet, even then, this crisis presented the doctors with an opportunity. For if the cause of the trouble was the toxoid, then ways might be found to change the procedure of its manufacture. If the cause lay, on the contrary, in their method of administration, that too might be changed.

We can imagine with what hesitancy they continued the tests, after the experience they had just been through. With any other test group, continuation would probably have been out of the question. In fact the doctors would have been lucky to get away from their patients with a whole skin. But this was a group of healthy, disciplined young men who had enlisted in their country's service for the purpose of taking risks. If the risks were worth the taking, if they would produce some facts of value to the Navy, there was no question but that they would take them.

So once again the injections began, with a new batch of toxoid, on the five hundred men who had not yet been given their second doses. One by one, they filed into the dispensary, and bared their arms to the surgeons' needles. But with the new toxoid, not a single one fell ill. No sore arms. No fevers. No malaise. No urticaria. No shock.

Hall and Hayden could breathe freely again. Their methods, at least, stood vindicated. And they had the answer to the rumors that were beginning to run around—the rumors that laid the blame on alum-precipitation. For many a doctor was beginning to say that alum-precipitated toxoid was unsafe. Yet here Hall and Hayden could prove that it wasn't all alum-precipitated toxoid that made trouble, but only this particular batch.

Still they wanted a final test that would prove their contention beyond a shadow of a doubt. And just then they received a new test group, the seven hundred and ninety-three students of the incoming class of 1939. These they proposed to test with the new toxoid, using it for both the first and the follow-up injections.

On the first series of injections they had just one, reaction case, a mild fever. So even the primary reactions of their preceding series, the ten men who reacted to the sensitizing dose, were not necessary. They too could be blamed almost entirely upon the "bad" toxoid rather than upon alum-precipitated toxoid as such. With the second injection on the new group, not a single plebe of all the 793 had any reaction whatever.

Now the doctors could turn to the remaining problem. What had been wrong with the bad batch? How could they prevent it from ever happening again? You couldn't ask the Navy or the Army to use a toxoid that you hoped wouldn't go wrong. You had to be sure that every last batch you ever produced would be just as good as the one you used on the Freshman Class of 1939.

So Dr. Hall and Dr. Hayden went to the laboratory that had produced their second "good" batch of toxoid. They watched it through every stage of its production. They saw how the alum was added to the toxin-antitoxin broth. They watched it in the centrifuge, where the alum was thrown by the whirling into the bottom of the jar, carrying with it the antigens and leaving the toxins behind. Then they watched the "washing." They saw salt solutions added to the alum precipitate. They saw the bottles go into an electrically driven churn, agitating the entire mass, mixing it thoroughly. Again and again the process was repeated, until the washing was thorough and complete and the final toxoid could be drawn off.

Then they went to the first plant they had dealt with, the one that had sold the "bad" batch. But everything was just the same. The same centrifuge. The same churn. The same washing.

That churn, in particular, was a honey. Everyone in the laboratory was proud of it. Their guide even boasted of the time it saved.

And there it was. They caught the phrase, "time it saved" and hung on to it for dear life. "What did you mean by that? Did you use another churn on the first batch you manufactured?" Hall demanded.

"Oh, no," came back the answer after much reference to the records. "We used hand agitation in the beginning."

For a moment the two officers didn't know whether to kill the man or kiss him. For now they had their answer. The trouble with the "bad" batch of toxoid came from inadequate washing. Something that should have been washed out had remained. Given adequate washing, this mistake need never occur again.

Though they had the answer the Navy wanted, though they could now safely proceed with total immunization throughout the service, Hall and Hayden had one more bit of sleuthing to do, if only to satisfy themselves. They wanted to find out what it was that had not been washed out of that trouble-making toxoid. Back to Annapolis they went and started to compare the good and bad batches. Both were exactly alike in all respects save one. The bad toxoid contained almost twice as much nitrogen as the good, 5.5% to

3.3%. It even contained more nitrogen than a standard sample of tetanus toxin, of the kind from which both batches were made.

That was nice to know, but what did it mean? They called in Dr. W. T. Harrison of the National Institute of Health and all three of them puzzled over the problem. Then someone got an idea. Whatever it was that contaminated the toxoid must be something with a high nitrogen content, so high that a little of it would raise the nitrogen rating of the whole batch by about two per cent. There was only one thing in the original broth that consisted of so much nitrogen, the proteins in the blood serum. They must be the villains.

So they began to give the standard protein tests to their toxoids. And they worked. The bad batch contained proteins. The good batch was protein-free.

Then they called in another worker, Chief Pharmacist P. S. Gault, and he worked out a new test. He took the alum-precipitated tetanus toxoid and dried it by evaporation. Then he treated it with concentrated hydrochloric acid, converting it into a water-soluble form. He followed the same procedure, of course, with both the good and the bad toxoids.

When he then put the good mixture into water, nothing happened. But when he put the bad actor into water solution, bang . . . the entire jar filled with a deep royal purple. Then he took some of the good toxoid and added some proteins deliberately. Again the water solution produced the same deep purple color.

With the Gault test they not only had the culprit, they also had a simple way of catching him. Even if proteins found some other defect in the process by which they might sneak into the toxoid, the Gault detector would show them up before the batch left the pharmaceutical factory.

Now at last Hall and Hayden felt that they had completely vindicated tetanus toxoid as such. Armed with this data they had no difficulty convincing the Navy medical authorities that tetanus inoculation should be made a standard Navy procedure.

The final proof of the value of immunization came a few months later, at Dunkirk. Unlike the French, the British had not made immunization in their army compulsory. They offered it to any man who wanted it and let it go at that. Most of the soldiers in the B.E.F. in France had accepted voluntary immunization. But about ten per cent had avoided it for one reason or another.

When the little British Army tried to stand off the Nazi blitzkrieg in the Dunkirk pocket, the bullets of course played no favorites. They hit the immunized and the un-immunized alike. And conditions were ideal for the development of tetanus. The wounded waited for hours, some for days, before they could be evacuated by small boats. They were carried through the surf to the pleasure craft that painfully and under a hail of Nazi bullets brought them across the channel.

Only after they reached hospitals in England was the time or opportunity found to administer antitoxin. No one was surprised, therefore, when out of the eighteen hundred men who had spurned immunization, eight developed tetanus. That was just about the normal incidence to be expected according to the averages of 1916 and 1917.

But if those averages were to hit with the same ferocity the sixteen thousand men who had been immunized, then seventy cases were to be looked for among the immunized men. Certainly anything less than that number could be considered at least a partial victory.

But nothing like seventy cases did appear. On the contrary, of all that sixteen thousand, worn and tired to a point where all resistance was gone—not a single one developed the slightest signs of tetanus.

The toxoid worked—100%.

That of course was the clincher. From that day on, any army that tolerated tetanus stood self-condemned as one that didn't care whether its men lived or died. The United States Army, which had been working on inoculation on an experimental basis for some time, quickly realized that experiments were no longer in order. Dunkirk had given the final answer. Early in the spring of 1941, the Surgeon General of the United

States Army signed an order adding tetanus toxoid to the list of compulsory inoculations to be given to every man inducted into service.

Today every soldier in our Army gets tetanus toxoid injections while he is still in training in the United States. If he is to be sent abroad, sometime in the preceding month he will be given an additional stimulating dose. At the end of every year he will get another such dose, at home or abroad. This is more than is actually necessary, but the Army is taking no chances.

Chapter VII

THE MINDSAVERS

IT happened near Bryansk. The Nazis had been pushing small groups at the Russian lines all day but they had gotten nowhere. They would send a squad of automatic riflemen around the little hill to the left and the hedge-hopping observation plane would spot them. The Russian snipers would each smoke a cigarette and when it was burnt down to the butt they knew that it was time to catch the Nazis as they came around the hill into the open. Then they'd pick them off, one by one, as they tried to cross the open field. Lieutenant Perfiliev would laugh when they came back to the dugout from these excursions. "Ten more blackbirds picked off the fence," he would say. His men always held their fire until he got the first Nazi; they figured that Perfiliev had a special score to settle because they all remembered his blue-eyed little sister and they also remembered the time they had found her body after the battle at Elets. Yes, they all had scores to settle, but Perfiliev had a right to priority on the first shot.

163

Towards evening, the Nazis brought up eight light tanks and when they came round the little hill all their infantrymen hid behind the slow-moving tanks. Badygin got one of the tanks with a grenade. The left tread was blown completely off so that all the frantic driver could do was to pivot around until they finished him off with another grenade. Someone from the company off at the far left got another tank. But the rest got through to the deserted village and the best the Russians could do was to close the line again and isolate the tank group. Perfiliev was mad all through, with that cold sort of madness that makes a man silent and thoughtful. "They'll hole up in the village for the night," he said to himself. "They'll think they're safe until morning. Well, we shall see. We shall see."

Perfiliev didn't ask for volunteers. He had tried that before and knew just what would happen. There was no sense in asking for volunteers when every man would step forward. Instead, he sent word down the line, and after a little while five squads came back to the dugout one by one. They waited till the moon had set, about ten o'clock. Then they worked back toward the village and waited again. At exactly ten-thirty a single shot echoed toward them from the front line and they knew that the men back there were all set against a relieving attack. From four sides, the squads came at the village to catch the tired Nazis off guard. They found the fools all together, quartered in the church, the tanks arranged around the building in a circle with one man guarding each. Perfiliev's orders were to get the tanks intact, if possible. Two men went for each machine, Indian fashion, and six of the ten tanks were taken before the men in the church caught on to what was happening. After that, it was a free for all, with Perfiliev leading his reserve squad right through the wide church doors.

The whole thing took perhaps fifteen minutes before quiet settled down again. Of one hundred and eight Nazis, sixty-six lay dead, thirty-four had been captured, ludicrously, in their flea-ridden underwear as they slept on the hard church benches. Eight were held, gagged, where they had been taken at their posts on the tanks. Perfiliev had turned toward the church door to see that everything was in order outside when a figure moved near the altar. A single shot rang out, then four more as the Russian guards aimed for the point from which the first flash had come, there in the dark nave of the building. The half-clad Nazi lurched over the altar, swayed and fell with a single thud to the floor.

When the men rushed to their lieutenant, they couldn't see at first where he had been hit. Then they found the wound, a small hole at the nape of the neck. Those who weren't needed to guard the prisoners gathered around, in a solemn circle, while a medical private was brought in. One quick look was enough.

"We'll have to get him to a hospital immediately," was all he said, as he closed the wound with a gauze pad and a bit of tape. There was practically no bleeding.

Four of the men lifted the lieutenant into one of the captured tanks and perched a man with the regimental flag astride its turret, so that no one would mistake it for what it had been an hour before. They eased the unfamiliar gears in gently and let it roll down the rough road to the rear as smoothly as they could. The sergeant who was left in command turned to the field telephone and put word through for an air ambulance.

And so Senior Lieutenant Perfiliev, who had had a score to settle and had settled it, was brought by plane to Moscow and rushed by ambulance to the Central Institute of Experimental Medicine, to the Nervous Diseases Clinic of Dr. Nikolai Ivanovitch Grashchenkov. They examined him under the X-ray fluoroscope and found that the bullet, which had entered at the nape of the neck, had passed straight through the entire left side of his brain and lodged in the left frontal region. Some hair and a piece of his hat had been carried in with the shot, contaminating the wound. Infection had begun to set in and an immediate operation was in order. But the watching physicians shook their heads. To get at that bullet would have required probing through the track of the wound, almost the whole length of the brain from back to front. Even with

Grashchenkov's skillful hands on the job, they might get the bullet but they would certainly spread the infection right through the whole track of the wound. The mere act of probing would mean destroying additional parts of the brain. Perhaps they might save the man, if they were lucky, but they would certainly destroy his speech centers and who knew what else in the process.

Grashchenkov was as silent as the rest. He turned the X-ray plates this way and that, shaking his head slowly. Then he smiled and turned to his chief nurse. "Prepare for an operation," he said, "and, Nana, stop worrying. I think we may yet save the young lieutenant."

The doctors moved off to wash up for the operation. The autoclave hissed as the nurses took the hot instruments from its shining maw. Perfiliev was wheeled in and placed onto the operating table, the small wound showing at the back of his neck. Then Dr. Grashchenkov tucked his head through the door that led from the surgeon's washroom. "No, Nana," he said, "I'll want him face upward." The nurses shook their heads, uncomprehendingly, then obeyed.

The watching surgeons and assistants wondered too when they entered the room. But their questioning stares changed to smiles of approval when Grashchenkov, taking a last look at the X-rays, picked up a scalpel and slit the skin of the forehead above the left eye.

With a trepaning drill he quickly made a small opening in the front of the lieutenant's skull. Then he cut through the dura, the inner membrane that envelops the brain. Less than a half inch below he found the bullet, removing it with a long-pronged forceps. Then he packed the wound with sulfathiazole and sewed up the dura. The bone was set back into place and the skin closed over the hole in the forehead.

A few weeks later a young man in a bright new uniform entered Dr. Grashchenkov's office. In crisp, clear Russian, Senior Lieutenant Perfiliev, who but for the man in front of him might never have talked again, addressed the surgeon. "Comrade Doctor," he said, "I'm going back to my regiment tomorrow. Before I go, I wanted to thank you. . . ."

Grashchenkov smiled and raised a deprecating hand in embarrassment, but the lieutenant wouldn't stop. "I wanted to thank you," he continued, "and to ask you a favor."

"A favor?"

"Yes, doctor. I wondered if you could let me have my bullet. My men would like so much to see my bullet."

Grashchenkov arose and put his arm around the young lieutenant's shoulder. Together they walked to a glass-fronted wall cabinet. There, lined up like so many soldiers on parade, were bullets of every size.

"It will spoil my collection," said the surgeon, "but I suppose, comrade, we can spare you one bullet."

Nikolai Grashchenkov is barely forty-one, yet he is recognized in the Soviet Union as one of their greatest specialists in the treatment of the brain and the spinal column. Nor do the Russians lack for skilled brain surgeons, except in so far as any army lacks for surgeons when its men stand up to the heaviest assault in history month after month. For it has been the policy of the Russian Army to train teams of specialists so that special surgeons and special hospitals can be set up, even near the front lines, to give the best possible care to the seriously wounded. The Chief Surgeon of the Red Army is, in fact, a brain specialist, Nicholai Nilovich Burdenko, a man whose peacetime activities have led non-Russians to think he must be several men bearing the same name. For Burdenko, the grandson of a serf and the son of a poor office clerk, has found time apart from his army duties to found and head the Soviet Central Neuro-Surgical Institute, to serve as President of the Medical Council of the People's Commissariat for Health, as Chairman of the All-Union Association of Surgeons, and as a Deputy to the Supreme Soviet of the U.S.S.R. It is as if our own Surgeon General were to take on the duties of a Congressman and still find time to double in brass as the President of the American Medical Association.

Burdenko is no youngster. He first saw action as a military surgeon during the Russo-Japanese War of 1903, receiving the Cross of St. George for tending the wounded under fire in the Far East. He again served his country during the World War and, after the revolution of 1917, took his place as one of the leading surgeons in the Soviet Union. In the Soviet-Finnish War, Burdenko again distinguished himself by establishing a surgical hospital only half a mile from the front lines, where soldiers with brain wounds could be operated upon. Before the establishment of this hospital, military field surgery practice called for brain operations far behind the lines because of the intricacy of such operations. By establishing a completely equipped surgical unit so close to the front, Burdenko and his associates saved the lives of hundreds of Red Army men and worked out techniques which have since saved many thousands more.

In the Soviet-Finnish campaign, brain-wound mortality was brought down to 13.9 per cent, less than half the best figure achieved in the last war by our own Dr. Harvey Cushing. Yet Burdenko and, for that matter, all the Russians readily acknowledge their debt to Cushing and model their techniques after those worked out by this, the greatest of all brain surgeons. It was Cushing, for instance, who insisted on early treatment of brain wounds, against all the precepts of the British and French, when he came to France in

1917. Cushing, too, was the leader in introducing specialized teams and particularly "brain teams" into military work. He trained scores of younger men for such specialization because brain operations call for a combination of stamina and dexterity which only a youngish man can provide over a long period of heavy service. How well the Russians have learned the lessons Cushing taught is shown by the constant references to the American which crop up in Soviet surgical literature. When a Soviet surgeon wants to say that he uses the best approved methods he writes, "using the Cushing technique."

Unlike the prophet of the proverb, Harvey Cushing is honored quite as much in the memory of his own country's surgeons as he is revered in Russia. Probably a good quarter of the brain surgeons of the United States have studied at one time or another under Cushing. Certainly none could pretend not to have studied his methods. For Cushing's techniques are the very bone and marrow of brain surgery, developed by a man who entered this specialized field when brain operations were an almost always fatal experiment and who left it studded with his pupils, the men who in turn have trained the younger men who came too late to witness the miracles of Cushing's work in 1918.

When, for instance, Gilbert Horrax, who worked with Cushing in France, proposed to set down the principles of treating war wounds of the brain as a guide for younger men, he told of the latest techniques, many of which the surgeons of 1918 could hardly have imagined. Yet it is significant to note that the majority of the diagrams that illustrate his text were labeled by Horrax as "modified from Cushing."

One of Cushing's most famous methods was developed for wounds in which a metal fragment has penetrated through the wall of the skull and lodged in the brain, usually carrying with it fragments of bone and sometimes other debris, such as hair or bits of clothing. The operation is also used for so-called *gutter wounds* in which the bullet fractures the skull without itself piercing or penetrating into the brain. In both cases a section of the brain will be reduced to a pulpy mass spotted with fragments of bone and debris.

Cushing's technique was to cut back the scalp in such a way that it could later be drawn over the wounded area and sewn together. The exposed section thus created was substantially larger than the fractured portion of the skull, large enough to permit the surgeon to drill four holes with a burr drill at the corners of a square surrounding the fracture. By connecting these holes by means of a bone-cutting forceps, the doctor may lift out the whole bony area intact with the intention of later replacing it as a unit. All this is done while the patient is under a local anaesthetic. General anaesthetics are avoided, wherever possible, in order to place the least possible strain on the patient's system and so that his co-operation may be secured when needed. Cushing, for instance, sometimes asked his patients to cough at this point in the operation. The strain served to eject some of the injured brain matter and, sometimes, some of the bone fragments or foreign matter as well. The brain itself is insensitive to pain, the anaesthetics being used to subdue the pain of the scalp, the bone-cutting and the inner membrane or dura.

With or without the aid of a cough, the surgeon next utilizes a soft rubber catheter or hollow probe to which is attached a suction device. Probing gently along the track of the wound, the doctor feels with the catheter for bony fragments and then uses gentle suction to draw them out on the end of his instrument. Where suction alone will not work, a delicate forceps is used to grasp the buried fragment. Gradually inserting the catheter further and further into the brain, the surgeon clears out the injured area, drawing up pulped brain tissue, blood clots, and foreign debris bit by bit.

All bone fragments must be removed. The metal fragment or bullet that causes all the trouble may sometimes be left in the brain, where its removal would involve more damage than its presence. Usually it is taken out, too. If possible a forceps is used to grasp it but when it lies too deep or when the wound track would have to be spread wide to give the forceps access, some surgeons use an ingenious combination of a common ten-penny nail and a magnet. The nail, after sterilization, is inserted into the wound until its rounded tip comes into contact with the steel slug. Then a powerful electromagnet is touched to the other end of the nail, protruding from the wound. All three metal bodies become one for the moment under the force of magnetism and the surgeon is enabled to remove the nail and the missile together.

Many a time in this war surgeons will thus follow the long, tedious yet ever-so-successful process "after the method of Cushing," cleaning the injured brain matter and its contaminating bone scraps, hair, and metal fragments out of the brain without destroying unnecessarily a single bit of uninjured brain. But wherever doctors have the facilities, as they usually have in the U. S. Army Medical Corps, the method will be somewhat modified. The change is one which vastly shortens the time required for the operation and, at the same time, cuts down the chance of the surgeon leaving some slight portion of injured matter or contamination to form later an infinitely troublesome and often fatal brain abscess.

The surgeon utilizes an electro-surgical apparatus such as Cushing would have given an arm for in the busiest days of 1918. This device, attached to a scalpel or other surgical instrument, uses an electric current to seal off each tiny blood vessel during the very second when it is cut. The bloody mess that once characterized an operation is thus eliminated. But even more important is the fact that electric cauterization seals off the healthy tissues against contamination from the infected portions of a wound. The surgeon can work speedily because he can remove large segments at once, without worrying about spreading infection.

The operative procedure is identical with that of Cushing until the dura has been cut back. Then the electro-surgical device is worked *around* the track of the missile or bone fragments. A wall, of sealed-off brain cells, is established like a cylinder on all sides of the wound. Within this tube of protection the surgeon is free to work quickly. He uses a strong suction to clean out the soft injured brain matter, blood clots, and other debris. But he takes care to use a metal sucking tube, to which he attaches his electro-cautery wires. Thus he sterilizes as he works.

Soon he has removed a core of tissue, including a very small amount of uncontaminated brain surrounding the track of the missile. Against the loss of this slight quantity of unhurt brain matter he balances the advantage of speedy work and the greater assurance which his new instrument gives against the spread of infection. As the core of tissue is removed, an assistant inserts a flat spatula into the wound, holding back the sides of the cavity. The entire area, down to the very depths of the wound, can thus be cleaned out under direct vision. The surgeon works with the sureness and precision that comes only with a clear view, gaining speed when every second counts, yet sacrificing nothing for the achievement.

In Cushing's day, the great fear of every brain surgeon centered about post-operative complications. Try as they would to remove all possible contamination and all the dead and dying tissues that would provide a home for infection, they could never be sure that some few germs would not remain in the wound. Their patients would seem to be on the road to recovery. Each day, as the doctors made their rounds, the soldiers would greet them with brighter smiles. But then, after three or four or five days, something would happen to some of their men. They would grow listless and begin to complain of headaches. Their temperatures would rise. Doctor would look at nurse and nurse would look at doctor. The more intuitive patient would see in these stares the death-sentence confession that infection had set in, infection which the doctors did not know how to fight. Sometimes they operated again. Sometimes they succeeded. But at best, the second bout with death took a terrible toll in additional brain matter lost to the patient.

Today the doctors have a weapon against the formation of brain abscesses and against the development of meningitis, the most deadly of the post-operative complications. Once the wound has been thoroughly cleaned out, the tract is filled with sulfanilamide pow-

der, enough to give a high local concentration, enough
to fight any few remaining germs to a stand-off. They
back this up with oral doses of sulfanilamide or sulfathiazole for a week or ten days, until the temperature
has returned to normal and stayed thus for a day or
two. Usually it works. Certainly the reports coming
from Pearl Harbor, where severe brain wounds were
numerous, have indicated a far lower incidence of
post-operative complications than ever could have
been hoped for during the last great war.

Soldiers with severe brain wounds in the past have
often recovered only to fall victim to epilepsy six
months or more after their injury. This was particularly true in cases in which some foreign body, usually
a metal fragment, was left within the brain because its
removal would cause too great an injury to the essential parts of the brain structure. Brain surgeons have
thus found themselves confronted by a sorry pair of
alternatives. They could remove the missile. If they
did this, they knew that they would destroy some fac-
ulty of their patient most essential to a full life. They
might leave him mute or sightless in one eye or par-
alyzed in some section of the body. Yet if they tried to
avoid this danger by leaving the bullet in place, the
soldier might fall into an epileptic convulsion six
months later that would herald a series of such attacks
leading to eventual death.

Today the rule seems to be developing as, "When

in doubt, leave it in." For anti-convulsive drugs, such as phenobarbital, have been developed to a point where epilepsy has lost its menace. The patients are given the drug three times a day, by mouth, and are taught to take it as a routine for at least a year. If epilepsy does develop, the drug controls it and the patient is enabled to go through life with no outward signs of the disease and no untoward effects. If no symptoms are noted after a year—and better surgery has cut the incidence of epilepsy to a new low—the use of the drug is gradually dropped.

Ralph Cloward, who treated a large number of brain injuries in Hawaii, was surprised to find that most of the men brought to him were conscious. "The majority of them," he wrote, "had not even been unconscious but were able to recall everything that had transpired from the time they were hit until they arrived at the hospital. This was the most surprising fact to the doctors who saw these cases. Patients with large gaping wounds in the frontal areas were found to be conscious, co-operative, rational and able to give their identifications. Most of the patients were in a state of mild shock but, aside from this, their normal physiologic functions did not appear to be altered materially."

The doctor's surprise reflects the change which has occurred in the treatment of all wounds, and brain wounds in particular, since the last war. For at Pearl

Harbor men were rushed straight to the hospitals and operated upon, almost invariably, within a few hours of injury. Thus the surgeons were able to observe and profit by the conditions which most World War I surgeons never met. For the earlier surgeons, with few exceptions, met their brain cases only in the rearward hospitals after many hours and sometimes days of painful evacuation. The conscious patient then was the exception, not the rule.

Pearl Harbor was, in other respects, not at all typical of the conditions under which most of our soldiers fight today. Caught off guard, the majority of the men had no head protection and consequently the incidence of brain wounds was much higher than it probably will be in the average planned action of the war. The "tin" helmet, when introduced in France in 1915, sharply cut down the incidence of brain injuries. The Russians report that, even where the helmet has been pierced and the brain reached, the severity of the wound is much reduced because the helmet breaks the force of the bullet or bomb fragment. Grashchenkov has reported that injuries to the skull or brain now vary from three to six per cent of the wounded, depending on the type of fighting and the nature of the terrain. This compares with an incidence for head wounds of from fifteen to twenty per cent in the last war.

Head armor has been vastly improved in recent

years and this improvement should have a pronounced effect on brain wounds. The American Army's "tin" hat has been discarded for a much deeper helmet of thicker and tougher metal, so designed as to provide protection from aerial missiles and bomb-bursts as well as from directly aimed rifle bullets. For naval anti-aircraft gunners, there has recently been issued a new type of helmet, much larger than any previously seen and designed to give a maximum of protection against strafing by hostile aircraft.

One would be indeed rash to dare to predict the number or even the percentage of fatalities from brain wounds to be experienced before the last shot of this war is fired. But already enough is known to let us set out some measures of the risks the average soldier will undergo.

We know that he will suffer less from bullet wounds of the head and more from splinters from shells and mines. The Russians report a drop in the percentage of head wounds caused by rifle bullets from more than fifty per cent in 1914-1918 to less than twenty per cent today. British experience confirms this trend and the, as yet, limited American experience seems to be following the same pattern.

We know that he will be better protected, by his helmet if he is an infantryman and by other forms of armor if he rides a tank or flies a plane, than were his predecessors in the last great war. This improved protection has likewise reflected itself in terms of both a shift in the proportion of wounds affecting the head and a lowering of the severity of head wounds. The mortality rate among the Russians in the Soviet-Finnish War was just under half that achieved by Cushing toward the end of World War I, less than a quarter of what it had been before Cushing came on the scene. Despite the adverse conditions induced by surprise at Pearl Harbor, brain-wound mortality there likewise cut well under the Cushing mark. Indications are that the Solomon Islands fighting has seen a maintenance and, in fact, an extension of this trend.

We also know, from the reports of hundreds of surgeons from the fighting countries, that methods of treatment are today far more effective in this department of military medicine. Given similar cases, the present-day surgeon should be able to save far more of his patients than his predecessors. Given wounds of lessened severity—as he now seems to be getting—the neuro-surgeon ought to be able to score an all time record for life-saving, brain-saving surgery.

Chapter VIII

THE JAPS GOT THE QUININE . . .

EVEN long after December seventh it was hard to realize, back in the States, that the war was already affecting every last one of us. It all seemed so far away. Names like Hongkong, Penang, Malacca, Sumatra, Timor, Bali, and Java, to most of us meant nothing more than the locale of travelogue movies.

Yet the Japs who plotted the conquest of Melanesia were not interested in capturing just the tourist-trade franchise. The little men who had planned this attack for forty years or more were after much more than palms and temple gardens. They intended to make us pay twice for every inch of territory they took, to cripple our ability to fight a global war by robbing us of vital sources of raw materials while forcing us, as the second payment, to divert other materials and endless effort in a hurried attempt to develop synthetics.

Did they take a tin mine in northern Malaya? They took ten thousand tons of gas, five thousand trucks, and a million man-days as well. For that is the price we must pay to reclaim tin from can collections once the mine is no longer ours. Did they conquer some thousands of acres of rubber trees, the production of which they could not possibly utilize for their puny motor industry? They took at the same time a million tons of Pittsburgh steel and Montana copper, ten million bushels of corn, and countless tons of fuel oil which we now have to divert from tanks and planes and explosives in order to make synthetic rubber. We were a self-sufficient nation, we thought. The jute and hemp we brought each year from the Far East were but a tiny fraction of all our imports, hardly worth counting against our domestic ability to produce. But the Japs who landed in the northern Philippines took more than a beachhead that December that seems so long ago. They took our principal source of naval rope and condemned us to incalculable effort and expense seeking new fibers throughout the Caribbean area.

But if our enemies had planned in Berlin and Tokio to finesse us neatly when it came to tin and rubber, they had one card to play that was intended to hurt us, not in two ways but in three. With this trump, they proposed to rob us of our accustomed source of supply, to send us on a wild scramble for a substitute, and to make us helpless meanwhile to fight back effectively. The key card the Nipponese intended to play was not to be found in the tin mines of the Malay States nor in the rubber of the Straits Settlements and Sumatra. It consisted of a few thousand acres of chincona trees set high on the uplands of Java, a few score of plantations that gave to those who controlled them a virtual monopoly of the only means which man has known, for three hundred years, for fighting malaria, the most widespread and consuming of all human diseases. With these acres our enemies gained an ally that would work for them on every tropical battlefield, an ally which—as they planned it—would make impossible for American troops ever to reconquer the vast, malaria-infected jungles of Burma, Malaya, the tropical isles, or the Philippines. Long before our men came into actual contact with the soldiers of Nippon, this ally would bring them down with chills and fevers of a disease that overnight converts good fighting men into enervated, listless hulks condemned, without quinine, to endless relapses and eventual death.

A beautiful, symmetrical plan, worthy of the minds that had planned and perfected the stab-in-the-back technique of warfare. A plan that almost worked. But one which is not working and will not work because, with fitting irony, the Japs' present allies gave us a pair of drugs that are potent against malaria and thus made it possible for the United States, under the driving impetus of national danger, to free itself of reliance upon the quinine plantations of Bandung on the Java plateaus.

We were not always dependent upon the Dutch

Quinine Syndicate. For the wondrous efficacy of the bark of the chincona tree was first discovered in Peru. The tales of its magic began to filter back to the old world three hundred years ago, long before doctors had the slightest idea of just what malaria was or how it spread. But though they were ignorant, until a few decades ago, of the nature of the chill-and-fever killer, doctors learned more and more about how to use the extracts of chincona bark to cure malaria or, at least, to end the crippling symptoms of the disease and make it possible for its victims to go on living and working until their next infection or relapse.

The tree grew wild in large areas of South America and, for many decades, it grew nowhere else. To keep the price up, each local despot of the Latin countries made the export of chincona bark a government monopoly. Each placed a complete interdict upon the export of the seed of the chincona tree. Yet so rapacious was their thirst for profits that they plundered their own forests, leaving the morrow to take care of itself. So much so that when the Dutch managed to get a single pound of seed, by stealth, to start their Java plantations, they soon found themselves in possession of a fabulously profitable quinine trade. As their carefully nurtured and cultivated plantations grew to bearing age, the last natural forests of South American chincona trees began to peter out. Natives had to be sent further and further into the hills to get any bark at all. Soon the low-cost plantation production of Java put the final seal on the South American trade and left the Dutch Kina Bureau in control of ninety-five per cent of the world's supply.

And so the United States and the United Nations were caught almost flatfooted when once it became clear that Java could not be held. Our Treasury Department had built up a stock pile sufficient for two years' peacetime consumption for the Western Hemisphere, more quinine than had ever been piled up before. But it was obvious from the very first that it would not begin to be enough for an army of millions, fighting in all the South Seas, perhaps in India, in China, certainly in the malarial lowlands of Europe.

"But doesn't our army know how to eliminate malaria?" you may well ask. "Haven't you heard that only thirty-one men in all our training camps in the last war died of malaria?" True, wonderfully true. Yet it is a very different thing to lick malaria at home and to fight it and the Japs and Germans at the same time, abroad. Our army chiefs knew what they were up against, in spite of their amazing victory over malaria in the last war. For that victory was a matter of drainage ditches and sanitation. We fought malaria by fighting the mosquitoes that spread the disease. We beat the rate of malarial infection among our soldiers down from 708 per 1,000 soldiers in 1902 to less than seven per 1,000 in 1927 and we've kept beating it down ever since.

But we did it on the home grounds, did it in our own sweet time, with every facility of community co-operation that an army can command from its own people. Our medical men knew that they would have no such simple task when our boats climbed the beaches of half a hundred foreign shores. There would be no time then for mosquito-killing campaigns.

Yet these doctors were not too worried. For there are other ways of fighting malaria besides killing mosquitoes. To understand these other ways, though, we will have to take a little course in the life history of the malarial parasite. To begin with, there are three kinds of malaria bugs, three single-celled animals known respectively as *Plasmodium Vivax, Plasmodium Malariae,* and *Plasmodium Falciparum.* Each differs from the other in some respects but all three have much in common, not the least of their similarities being the fact that they make you miserably sick when they get into your blood stream.

These plasmodia have a complicated life cycle. Let us start to follow it by watching a mosquito biting a man who has malaria. If it is one of several varieties of anopheles mosquitoes he will suck up infected blood containing malarial parasites. Some of these, the asexual *schizonts,* will die off in the mosquito's body. But a few will prove to be *gametocytes,* male and female parasites. These will breed within the insect's stomach. The fertilized female cell will bore into the stomach wall of the happy, oblivious mosquito. A cyst will form in the body cavity of the mosquito, growing until it matures and bursts. Then it will liberate, within the anopheles, a swarm of new parasites, millions of them. These will find their way into the salivary glands of the mosquito and thus the little dive bomber will be re-armed, ready to strike down another victim and inject him with a new lethal dose of malaria.

Once they get into man, the new malaria bugs begin to develop. The parasites bore into the red blood cells. Each picks a cell for itself, nests comfortably, and proceeds to divide into a series of from fifteen to twenty spores. When the spores are fully formed, the blood cell is ruptured and the new plasmodia go their way, looking for new red cells to conquer and destroy. Thus, by repeated cycles, the organisms multiply with extreme rapidity unless something interrupts their growth.

Plasmodium Vivax goes through its cycle in forty-eight hours. *Plasmodium Malariae* takes seventy-two hours per generation. *Plasmodium Falciparum* matures in from twenty-four to forty-eight hours. With the completion of each cycle, at the time when the growing parasites burst their blood-cell hosts, the body goes through a typical malarial paroxysm of chills, fever, and sweat. If the attack is light enough for nature eventually to fight it off, the victim survives but is so depleted in red blood cells that he is incapable of strenuous effort for a long time. If the attack is strong, the parasites breed until they conquer the blood, rob it of so many red cells that the victim dies. Every year, throughout the world, eight hundred million people suffer from malaria. Every year, three million or more die. And the disease is toughest on those who have not lived in malarial regions before, those who, like our soldiers, will get it for the first time.

While the sexless parasites are breeding and growing in the red cells, a few mature without splitting. These are the sexual types—the gametocytes—growing and waiting for a mosquito to carry them off. They don't cause much trouble in the human body, since they don't "eat" red blood cells. Instead, it is their function to carry on the cycle, to infect the next mosquito so that he can in turn infect the next human victim.

Now it becomes clear why killing mosquitoes, anopheles mosquitoes, is effective in ridding a region of malaria. For unless the mosquito can play its part in the cycle, the life history of the malarial parasite is interrupted. But there are two troubles with mosquito control programs. For one thing, they are extremely expensive. The federal and state governments have spent untold millions of dollars in digging drainage ditches, oiling swamps, and screening houses and barns in our southeastern states, yet the incidence of malaria has been hardly cut at all, simply because the region is too vast for the program to do much more than scratch the surface. In great swampy areas, the problem literally defies solution by these methods. Yet conditions in the continental United States are nothing as compared with the jungles of the Caribbean, South America, Burma, Malaya, and many other areas throughout the world.

Even more difficult than that, though, is the problem of synchronizing mosquito elimination with military activity. For you cannot institute much more of an anti-mosquito program than is represented by the use of nets and net sleeping-tents in any area you haven't thoroughly conquered. Certainly you cannot begin to apply large-scale drainage programs while the fighting front is skipping from island to island. Every time you conquer a new region, you acquire a native population teaming with malaria parasites, ready to give each new crop of mosquitoes a new dose of plasmodia. And neither mosquitoes nor malarial parasites draw any distinctions of race, color or creed.

It is for this reason that our army, and all others for that matter, have always planned upon interrupting the cycle of malaria at some other point when fighting in the field. That is why the conquest of the chincona tree plantations seemed, at first, more important to the Mikado than all the rubber trees in the world. For, until recent years, there was no other drug that could interrupt the malaria cycle and, until right now, no country could produce enough of the two present alternative drugs to supply anything like a large army in the tropics. Unfortunately for the Japs, however, it looks as if we'll get by. In fact, we'll probably get by handsomely.

Our first stroke of good fortune came in the early nineteen-twenties. It came, of all places, from the laboratories at Elberfeld-Wuppertal, the laboratories of the great Interressen Geselschaft Farbenindustrie, the German dye trust. Just why the Germans went after malaria was at first hard to figure. They had practically no malaria in their own country. They had lost all of their colonies. Yet go after malaria they did, possibly because in this, as in other things, they possessed the foresight that comes to those who wait and prepare only for the day when they shall conquer the world.

They had so little of the disease in Germany, that they couldn't gather together enough malaria victims to give their doctors good working samples at the start. But even then, as far back as 1925, some German industrialists knew that they wanted to be free of dependence upon all foreign materials when once they started on the road of conquest—and that included the Dutch monopoly, quinine. So they built aviaries and stocked them with canaries, thousands and tens of thousands of canaries. For canaries, though they never caught human malaria, did get infected by a similar parasite. They could be cured by quinine and it took just about as much quinine, per ounce of body weight, to do the trick on a canary as it did on a man.

Then the Germans began to analyze the chemistry of quinine, an extremely complicated drug. Soon they tried to imitate it synthetically and failed miserably. Nature was able to do something in forming the bark of the chincona tree that not even the master chemists of I. G. Farben were able to accomplish. Next, they turned to making something like quinine; anything as long as it would work. Along about 1925 they came up with a drug that seemed to do the trick. In fact, it did more than quinine would do. It not only killed the asexual form of the parasite—as quinine did —but it also rid the canaries of the male and female sexual types. Here, at last, it seemed, they had a way of really breaking the malarial cycle. For quinine broke it only in respect to the individual being treated for the disease. It killed the bugs that made the victim sick, but it left the other parasites waiting for the first handy mosquito to pick them up and carry them, vastly multiplied, to infect another victim. But plasmochin, as they called the new drug, rid the canaries of both types of parasites. Man had bested nature after all.

So it seemed, until they sent some of their doctors to Spain, where human malaria was rife enough to give them plenty of patients. Then they found that their new drug was a wonder-worker indeed—but not quite the miracle drug they thought it to be. It killed off the male and female gametocytes of human malaria just as it did the avian types. But against the asexual variety, the parasite that made you *sick* of malaria, the new drug was almost entirely ineffectual. As far as human malaria was concerned, all they turned out to have was a drug that might supplement quinine, if you could induce people to use it. That was hardly what they had been after and the whole project almost came to a dead stop.

Then the Germans went to work again, hitching their research wagon to the thin lead provided by the fact that acridine, a yellow coal-tar dye in no particular way like quinine, did have a lethal effect on trypanosomes, the parasites that caused sleeping sickness. It was a far cry, for these parasites had very, very little in common with the plasmodium of malaria. But it was all they had to go on, so on they went. After repeated failures, they found themselves wandering farther and farther away from their starting point, acridine, but nearer and nearer to a drug that would out-quinine quinine. Finally they worked up something with the astounding chemical name of "di-hydrochloride of 3-chloro-7-methoxy-9-(1 methyl-4-diethyl-amino) butylamino acridine." They called it atabrine, but what you called it didn't matter much. The fact was that it worked, faster, more thoroughly, and more permanently than quinine ever had.

Atabrine destroyed the asexual forms of the malaria parasite. When the victim suffered from *Plasmodium Vivax* or *Plasmodium Malariae,* the drug usually destroyed the sexual gametocytes as well. When dealing with *Plasmodium Falciparum,* the parasite most common in the malarial regions of the Far East, doctors usually have to fall back upon plasmochin to supplement atabrine. But used alone, or used in conjunction with its sister drug, atabrine has completely out-distanced quinine in almost every respect.

As soon as the drug was introduced in 1933, reports began to come in from every malarial region in the world, reports which, had they been made singly, would probably have been condemned as the vaporings of doctors who had a touch of malarial fever themselves. But the very weight and number of these documents seemed to answer all doubts. One of the first reports concerned a study made by the famous British malariologist, Colonel S. P. James. He and his associates infected seven selected volunteers with the same strain of *Plasmodium Falciparum* by bites from the same experimentally infected mosquitoes. Two of the patients were treated with quinine. They took two grams daily, a fairly heavy dose, for twelve and fourteen days, respectively. Yet they were still uncured.

Then they were given a five-day course of atabrine, three pills a day, and the infection was eliminated.

The other five patients started right off with the atabrine course. Every day, each of them took a total of three-tenths of a gram of the new drug. At the end of five days, all five of them were completely cured. Again and again these tests were made, on new groups of volunteers, and each time atabrine cured the infection in five days, bringing the chills and fever to an end usually by the second night.

In Malaya, Dr. A. L. Hoops tested atabrine in 1933 on 317 natives and Europeans. After cure, 253 of his patients were kept under continued observation and, of these, only ten suffered later relapses. Previous experience with quinine showed a relapse rate more than twice as great. After that, quinine was dropped entirely by the large rubber estates in the Malacca region in favor of atabrine. The number of hospital admissions dropped each year. Vomiting, frequent with quinine, became a rare occurrence. Fevers and chills usually disappeared by the third day. Even pregnant women and those reactive to quinine were able to take the new drug without trouble.

In the Punjab Province of India, Brevet-Colonel F. M. Lipscomb treated nearly seven hundred British soldiers with atabrine, sometimes supplementing this treatment with a later course of plasmochin. Only 8.6 per cent suffered later relapses as against a 25 per cent relapse rate when quinine was the only drug available.

Soon the reports came tumbling in. In the Philippines Dr. P. F. Russell wrote of atabrine as the best anti-malarial drug available. At the United Fruit Company Hospital in Santa Marta, Colombia, doctors wrote of the "spectacular results of curing all patients in one week or less." From India, Burma, England, Rumania, Panama, Cuba, and from Georgia, Tennessee, Arkansas, and Florida, the reports all varied in detail, but all agreed on the one essential group of facts: fewer relapses, quicker cures, reduction in the death rate, reduction of complications. Abortions among malarial mothers, once the rule with quinine, began to be a rarity when atabrine was the routine drug. Against all this, the worst that could be said of atabrine was that it had a tendency to discolor temporarily the skin of those who took it—as if a jaundiced look, with no other bad effects, was any price at all to pay for freedom from malaria!

With all these records of speedy cures, it was natural that army men and health authorities should begin to think that possibly here was the means of eliminating malaria from whole regions. For atabrine killed not only the asexual forms of all three malarial parasites, it also killed the disease-spreading sexual forms, of two of the three types. And plasmochin killed the male and female gametocytes of the third type. Seemingly they had everything necessary for prevention as well as for cure.

One of the first things they learned, however, was that they couldn't safely combine atabrine with plasmochin. They tried that and they found that the two drugs, given together, were far more toxic than either given separately. But even this minor difficulty was soon eliminated by the simple device of giving a course of atabrine, waiting two days while the body eliminated the drug, and then starting the plasmochin treatment.

There were a few other illusions that had to be swept out of the way. Before the days of atabrine, there were many physicians and innumerable laymen who believed that quinine was an effective prophylactic. Tradition had it that if a person in a malarious place would take a dose of quinine at sunset and another at sunrise, all the parasites injected by a mosquito which bit them during the night would be killed and they would not suffer malaria. To demolish this strange belief, Colonel James, as Advisor on Tropical Diseases to the British Ministry of Health, made a series of tests. He recorded the temperature charts of people who took quinine shortly before being bitten by mosquitoes and continued to dose themselves for ten days. He found, as he had expected, that the quinine had no effect in preventing or delaying the malarial attack.

Then he thought he would put atabrine to the same test. This time he used three series of patients. Some took no drugs, some took quinine, and some took atabrine. Of the first two groups, every patient had an attack of the disease after the usual incubation period. But, with the last group, not a single one fell ill. Seemingly, Colonel James had shown just how to eliminate all malaria. But when he tried the same trick against other strains, it did not work quite as certainly and completely. The parasites were just a bit too subtle to be dismissed so easily. Yet James did succeed in showing that atabrine was better able to protect against at least some forms of malaria and, most important, he laid at rest the dangerous delusion that quinine could be used prophylactically.

But the real credit for the development of prophylaxis must go to a group of Americans. They have all worked on the gametocyte theory, figuring that if they could eliminate malaria carriers, people who supplied the mosquitoes with male and female parasites, they could reduce the incidence of the disease to zero by eliminating the source of the infection.

The first of these was Dr. Daniel L. Seckinger of the Georgia Department of Public Health. In 1933, aided by two Negro practical nurses, Dr. Seckinger invaded dank, undrainable Calhoun County, a region so racked by malaria that over eighty per cent of all school children had a blood index positive for the disease in the fall of 1932. The population was almost entirely Negro. Whites had moved away year by year, leaving the rich land to be feebly worked by a rural population of thirteen hundred and twenty-five spread over an area of more than fifty square miles. Starting in May, the doctor from Atlanta and his two aides began to give their atabrine and plasmochin pills to all the people in six of the eight school districts. In two districts, identical in every respect, including malarial incidence and severity, some four hundred people were reserved as a control group.

To everybody in their six selected districts, they gave a small dose of plasmochin three times a week. To anyone who actually developed the symptoms of malaria—and there were plenty of these—they gave the regular atabrine course of three pills a day for five days. Just to make doubly sure, they took blood tests every month and dosed all those who showed a positive blood smear, even though the symptoms of clinical malaria might not be present, with the five-day atabrine treatment. By the end of the malaria season in 1933 there was no doubt of the efficacy of their drugs. In the control area, over sixty per cent of the people had had the disease during the season. The rate of infection in the six treated districts was only 10.6 per cent.

Then in October, Dr. Seckinger kept his promise to those in the untreated areas and gave every man, woman, and child an atabrine course. This was bad science, for it affected his control group so that future studies would be thrown out of line. But though it may have been bad science it was good medicine and Daniel Seckinger felt that this was the least he might do for the people who had helped him all year despite their ague and fever.

Then came 1934, the worst malaria year in generations in that area of Georgia. The death rate in surrounding regions mounted to 109 per 100,000. But in the treated area there was so little malaria, comparatively, that the people in all the adjoining counties began to talk of Calhoun as the place where malaria didn't exist. Which was an exaggeration, true enough, but not so much of an exaggeration at that. For in the control areas, where only the end-of-season atabrine course had been given in 1933, the incidence of malaria was still halved. It started low, and even at the peak of the season, it never topped 28.8 per cent. The results in the areas that had been thoroughly treated with both atabrine and plasmochin were even more astonishing: only 8.8 per cent of malaria showed up by October, 1934.

That was the year when Dr. M. E. Winchester took office as Health Commissioner of another Georgia county, Glynn. To say that he "took office" is hardly correct. The office was thrust on this country doctor, but once he took up the burden, he looked around him and he knew that his main work must be malaria. As records go in Georgia, Glynn County wasn't bad. Its malaria rate seemed to be low. But Dr. Winchester knew how records could lie, knew that there was practically no malaria on the rich coastal islands where the big estates and clubs were located, nor in the well-drained and thoroughly oiled sections around Brunswick. But he also knew about the backwoods of Glynn County where a thousand families worked a region so desolate and water-soaked that drainage was unthought of, where during the bottom of the malaria year, in February, 1934, he found forty per cent of the people with a history of malaria the previous summer.

Dr. Winchester went up to Atlanta where he sat around and talked things over with the State Health Commissioner, Dr. Abercrombie, and with Dan Seckinger. Then he went over to the Federal Relief people and talked some more with them. When he finally went back to Glynn County, he brought with him seven unemployed nurses and all the atabrine pills he could tote. Then he and his nurses lined up every person in the test area who proved blood positive in the malaria survey and dosed them with atabrine. But they went beyond that. They dosed every member of the family, even if only one had had malaria. Altogether they gave their fifteen pills to 1,369 people out of a total of some two thousand in the area. And then, in autumn, when malaria should have been at its peak, they retested the blood of everybody. Instead of the original seven per cent positive they had scored on their first tests in February, they now found a mere eight-tenths of one per cent.

Of their 1,369 atabrine cases, ninety per cent had used quinine before. Yet a majority of them had had to use it over and over, reporting a history of repeated attacks. But that first summer of Winchester's experiment, he had only fifty relapses and these were brought around by a second fifteen-pill course. The schoolteachers, who once sent half their classes home some days, could hardly believe their eyes or their record books. In all that school season, not a single child had to be sent home with chills and fever. Finally, Doc Winchester had the pleasure of signing the county mortality table for the year. It gave him a kick to know that Abercrombie would understand why Glynn County reported eight malaria deaths in 1933 and had a big black zero on the same spot on the 1934 chart.

The State Health Commissioner did more than read this report. This time he took the train and went to ask a favor of Winchester. When the malaria season rolled around in 1935, Winchester was on special assignment of the Georgia State Board of Health conducting a new experiment in prophylaxis in the Harris Neck section of McIntosh County. Harris Neck can only be inadequately described as a swamp country

Tobacco Road. He examined the 244 Geechee Negroes who constituted the population of his malaria-ridden neck in the woods. All who were found to harbor malarial parasites were given the regular five-day treatment of atabrine. By this time there was no question that atabrine would rid the body of malarial schizonts. Winchester was after something bigger than that. To prove his theory he had to be sure that he started off the season without any malaria carriers.

Once he'd cured them all, he secretly divided the entire group into two evenly matched halves. To the family on every alternate farm, he gave one pill of atabrine every day from May 15 to the end of October. To every other family he gave little yellow pills also, but these pills were nothing but a very mild laxative. That fall not a single member of any of the atabrine families had shown any signs of malaria. But of the 120 persons in the control group, the people who took the inert yellow pills, 58 came down with the chills.

That pretty much proved that atabrine was, to say the least, the best prophylactic against malaria they had yet found. But to make doubly sure that this was not some freak of chance, Winchester repeated the same test for the next two years, using a somewhat larger group. He had to enlarge his test group because this time everyone in Harris Neck insisted upon being put in the prophylactic group. In order to get a control

unit he had to count in the people of the equally malaria-ridden adjacent country. Malaria in Georgia was
worse in 1936 than the year before, yet again, not a
single case turned up in his prophylactic group. Winchester expected this, but even he was somewhat surprised to find that the malaria rate fell to exactly half
of what it had been the year before in the control
group.

The next year there was a repeat performance, only
again the control group too showed a dropping off.
This time the malaria rate among this group came to
only 16.9 per cent. By then they knew their answer.
They had just as many mosquitoes around Harris Neck
as ever before. But they had infinitely fewer people
infecting those mosquitoes. Winchester, who just
started out as a plain county health agent, ended up
by proving that the new drug was not only a cure but
a preventive. To top that off, he found he had also
proved that if enough people used it as their individual protection, they ended up by protecting everybody
all around as well.

Since that time, the twin drugs have been subjected
to hundreds and hundreds of other tests, all over the
world. Not all have been quite as hundred-per-cent
certain as Winchester's Georgia experiments, for malaria is a different sort of devil in different countries.
The tropics present conditions far more difficult for
would-be malaria-conquerors, for in equatorial re-

gions there is no single mosquito season. Instead new crops of mosquitoes mature, get infected, transmit the infection, and lay their eggs all the year around. Native populations, in many sections, are adjusted to malaria, if you can use that term to characterize a condition that condemns everyone to an early death. The disease is not epidemic but endemic. Everyone—or almost everyone—is a carrier of the mosquito-infecting gametocytes. Naturally, under such circumstances, even in peacetime, the prophylactic use of the new malarial drugs is a far more difficult procedure and one far less likely to provide the clear-cut results achieved in Georgia and other southern states.

The Army and Navy are well aware of the menace of malaria. Army doctors have long been in the forefront of anti-malarial studies in the Canal Zone, in Cuba, in the Philippines, and, more recently, in all our new island bases. The non-medical military men, too, know what malaria can do to an army if the doctors aren't given every chance to fight the disease. They cannot forget, for instance, the British division sent into Greek Macedonia during the last war. These troops had been no more than two weeks in the country when they began to go down with malaria at a rate exceeding one hundred a day. Within a year, in this single division of some fifteen thousand men, there were thirty thousand cases of malaria. Every man, on the average, had the disease in acute form at least twice. The next year they had seventy thousand cases, an average of more than four infections per man!

No wonder then that the Army has taken drastic steps to insure an adequate supply of anti-malarial drugs, adequate on a scale far greater than ever contemplated before. Five days after the declaration of war, the use of quinine for any but anti-malarial purposes was prohibited. New facilities for the production of atabrine and plasmochin were put on the preferred list immediately after Pearl Harbor. Reserve stocks have been built up in quantities that make former production look minuscule. Just how large these quantities are is confidential military information, but that they are large is no secret. The sole producer in this country of both drugs was a firm having close connections with the German dye trust. But since war was declared, that firm has operated under the direct orders and control of the Alien Property Custodian and thus, in effect, the government is producing its own anti-malarial drugs.

The methods used by the Army and Navy in fighting malaria must vary with each situation. In permanently located bases overseas, principal reliance is laid upon sanitation measures which eliminate the local vectors, the mosquitoes which transmit the disease. When preparing to enter infected regions, it is probable that some form of prophylactic dose will be utilized, such as an atabrine pill daily for every man. This course may be continued as a precautionary measure indefinitely or it may be dropped as soon as sanitation measures can be adequately installed. Certainly, whenever malaria does break out, our men will not stop with the mere relieving of the symptoms of the individual, important as that may be. Carriers of the gametocytes will be eliminated by plasmochin treatment before being released from medical department supervision.

Undoubtedly, our armed forces and those of our allies, will find it necessary to extend these treatments to part, if not all, of the native populations they encounter. For prophylactic measures among our own men alone will avail little if the regional mosquitoes are constantly being re-infected by the infected blood of native carriers. Thus it may turn out that the scourge of war now visiting the bewildered denizens of Africa and the South Seas may yet prove a boon in disguise, since it may leave wide malarial regions free—or at least freer—of malaria than they have ever been in the past.

Those of our men who do get the disease will undergo the regular fifteen-pill treatments. Most of them will be fit to return to duty within a few days, little more affected by their experience than if they had incurred a severe cold. But when they move from region to region, and particularly before they return to the States, they will be re-examined and re-treated to eliminate the possibility of relapses which often occur as a result of moving from a malarial district to one where malaria is rare or unknown.

Chapter IX

TAKING THE TERROR OUT OF WAR'S
WORST WOUNDS

ON the shores of Lake Ladoga there once stood a Grand Duke's summer palace, converted into a sanitarium to which the City of Leningrad used to send its children for medical observation. The kids loved the place, with its rolling lawns leading down to the great lake, busy with chugging tugs and packed excursion steamers. The lawns cut a gash through the otherwise unbroken pine forest and the smell of pine needles was everywhere.

Then one day, the sound of guns was heard to the north. A pall of smoke rose on the Karelian Isthmus and drifted lazily across the lake. A long line of busses drove up to the sanitarium and stood in a ring in the snow while the children were bundled into their warmest clothes. As the laughter-filled cars made off towards the south, they met a longer line of trucks bearing the insignia of the Red Army Medical Corps and loaded down with surgical supplies. The Russo-Finnish War was on and the Grand Duke's palace was to become a Special Thoraco-Surgical Hospital.

Soon a squad of men with tractors was clearing and smoothing the deep ice of the lake, forming runways for the ski-fitted planes that would bring the wounded down from the fighting in the north. The ski-pull, which the children had so enjoyed as its chugging gasoline motor pulled them up the long slopes, was converted into an evacuation device, equipped with improvised closed cars, so that the injured could be loaded directly from the planes on the lake shore and carried, smoothly and speedily, up to the hospital on the top of the hill.

There, for the next four months, a special group of surgeons—all chest specialists—worked under the direction of Professor B. E. Linberg. By ambulance and, mostly, by plane, there were brought to the hospital 972 seriously wounded men, unselected except for the fact that they had chest injuries and had survived to reach this hospital. If anything, the conditions under which these men had fought, in the forty-degree-below-zero blizzards of the Finnish winter, made their condition somewhat more serious, their chance of successful recovery somewhat less. Not that those chances had ever been too good. For chest wounds have traditionally been considered among the most frequently fatal of all war wounds.

If these 972 men had fought in the British Army during the Crimean War, 79.2 per cent of them would have died. If they had served in our own Civil War,

62.6 per cent would have failed of recovery. If they had been in the Russian Army of the first World War, death would have taken from thirty to forty per cent of those who reached a hospital, and many of course among these 972 would not have lived to find a hospital bed. Even if they had fought with the British in the last war, 27.5 per cent would have died. Twenty-four per cent of the hospitalized American wounded of this type in World War I, died of their injuries. In all the wars from which statistics are available, only once did this figure of chest-wound fatalities fall below fifteen per cent and then only in the Boer War, where a far better climate and the predominant use of light arms combined to make for a very special, non-typical situation.

But at the Special Thoraco-Surgical Hospital outside of Leningrad, death was induced to take a holiday. Of nearly a thousand men for whom its hand had reached, only twenty-nine in all died. Instead of seventy, sixty, or even twenty-five per cent, the death rate was cut to three per cent. And twelve of those suffered not merely from chest wounds but from combined wounds of the chest and other regions.

Here was no mere quantitative change, no mere cheating of death by some neat surgical trick, important though such tricks may often be. For the Russian figures represent, more than anything else, the deliberate, planned application of all our new knowledge of thoracic surgery to the problems of warfare. Professor Linberg and his fellow surgeons were given no carefully selected group to work upon; these men were no worse off and certainly no better off than the average of the severely wounded. But Linberg was given every last advantage in transport, equipment, and facilities. And he added to these the further advantage of a team of trained chest specialists utilizing the best techniques his country had worked out in twenty years. It was from all these elements combined that he brewed the formula that so signally defeated death. Thus, the events of the winter of 1939-1940 on the windswept shores of a frozen lake were not merely a Russian victory; they showed quite clearly that we or any other nation could achieve similar results by the same methods. Chest wounds, once the most fatal of all war wounds, have been put in their place.[1]

Before we can get a clear picture of just what the Russian formula was, we will have to get a better idea of the structure and functioning of the chest. In point of fact, the lack of such a clear understanding was one of the major causes of high chest-wound mortality in

[1] It should be understood, of course, that in all the figures cited above, we refer to hospitalized chest wounds. Death rates, on the battlefield, have always run high and are still high. Little can be done for such causes of almost instant death as wounds of the heart or of the major blood vessels. But the Russian figures are, if anything, loaded a bit against the doctors, for they include many men who would once have died on the way to the hospital and who now reach the surgeon because of motorized or airplane evacuation. These border-line cases make the lowering of the death rate all the more notable.

earlier wars; doctors either adopted a conservative wait-and-see attitude from fear of their own ignorance or entered the chest only to hurt rather than help the patient. This was true even during the first years of World War I.

Military surgeons, in 1915 and 1916, relied on their experience with chest wounds in the Boer War, where it had been found better to leave most such injuries to the natural processes of cure. It was only in 1917, after the vastly different conditions of the Western Front had caused thousands of deaths from wounds that nature just wouldn't heal unaided, that the French and British medical services began to apply the general rules of surgery to chest wounds. In July of that year, a meeting of consulting surgeons drew up a memorandum which was communicated as a guide to all medical units. Immediately after this and for the rest of the war, the death rate from chest injuries was cut substantially.

The importance of early and decisive surgical intervention for most chest wounds becomes apparent when we view the structure of the chest. To begin with, we have a bony cage, formed by the ribs and the backbone. At the bottom of this cage and projecting upward in the center, is a thin, muscular wall, the diaphragm, which separates the chest from the abdomen. The space above the diaphragm is in turn divided in two by a vertical wall, the mediastinum. Inside the two large cavities thus formed lie the lungs, pulling like evenly balanced springs on each side of the central wall. The lungs are, of course, partly hollow, spongy and elastic, so much so that they would collapse except for one thing: the pressure of the air within them. Any contraction away from the chest wall immediately sets up an area of vacuum or negative pressure between the lung and the surrounding chest cavity.

Thus we see that one of the first consequences of a penetrating chest wound is to disturb this pressure relationship. The tendency to collapse, which has always been balanced by the negative pressure around the lungs, now can have full play once air is admitted through the wound. Instead of a negative pressure, we have equal air pressure on either side of the lung, the pressure of the ordinary atmosphere. The lung collapses just like a toy balloon, drawing upward to the bronchial tube to which it is attached. This condition, known as pneumothorax, is not necessarily harmful. In recent years, in fact, it has become common practice to induce it artificially, by injecting air through a needle into the chest cavity, to rest the lungs of tubercular patients.

When pneumothorax is caused by a bullet or shell splinter the surgeon must first of all guard against infection. The greatest danger, however, lies in a ragged chest wound that acts as a valve. For then, every attempt by the patient to exhale draws air through the wound, air which cannot be expelled when the lung tries to fill up again. This *tension pneumothorax* sets up an increasing pressure in the wounded half of the chest which, sooner or later, tends to force the central partition—the mediastinum—to the other side, where it will encroach upon the breathing capacity of the remaining lung.

To defeat this condition, and to ward off infection, it is essential that the "sucking" wound of a pneumothorax be closed at the earliest opportunity. For this purpose, all armies now provide their medical-aid men with one or another form of special dressing for sealing an open chest wound against the passage of air. Such bandages can easily be improvised and should always be available in one form or another. In Spain, where even the most elementary surgical necessities were often lacking, the occlusive bandage consisted of several thicknesses of blotting paper. The made-up bandages were sterilized in the autoclaves of the Number I (or nearest-the-front) Hospitals and carried by the Battalion Aid Troops. They were applied to the open wounds and sealed in place by layers of adhesive plaster. Then the bandage was marked with a distinctive cross to indicate that it should not be removed under any circumstances until the operating table was reached.

A second consequence of wounds of the chest is

known as *hemothorax* or hemorrhage into the chest cavity. Here, bleeding vessels, either of the chest wall or of the lung itself, gradually fill the base of the chest cavity with fluid blood which usually clots little if at all. If the bleeding is from the lung, one of nature's compensatory mechanisms usually holds it to minor limits, for the collapse of the lung tends to close off the bleeding vessels and stop the hemorrhage. When the bleeding, as is more frequently the case, is due to injury of blood vessels in the chest wall, a very substantial amount of blood may gather. Hemothorax combines the dangers of pneumothorax with some additional ones of its own. Like any hemorrhage, it leads to severe shock unless arrested. The presence of blood, particularly fluid blood, within the area of the wound, is an open invitation to infection. And the blood serves to displace the chest organs and prevent the injured lung from again assuming its proper place in the breathing procedure.

The Russians have somewhat modified earlier procedures in dealing with hemothoracic wounds. For one thing, they felt that the earlier policy of waiting for some days before removing the gathered blood was ill advised, since it delayed natural recovery processes and increased opportunities for infection. Thus, as soon as shock had abated and the patient's condition allowed, usually on the third or fourth day, Linberg and his associates would drain away this blood, using a wide-bore needle to pierce the chest wall and draw off the blood. As against the fear, expressed by other surgeons, that infection would occur as a consequence of early removal of the gathering blood, the Russian experience showed a very low incidence of infection. Of 96 cases of hemothorax only two became infected. Not a single one died. This they ascribe in large measure to one innovation of their procedure. Linberg not merely withdrew the blood but he combined this operation with an irrigation of the chest cavity with a mild antiseptic. Thus they actively fought off the possibility of spreading infection.

The Russian experience was not without its disclosures of weakness in the surgical procedures. Thus it was found that many of the front-line surgeons knew too little of the anatomy of the chest wall. In about one-quarter of all the cases of pneumothorax, which had been sutured to effect closure, by doctors at reception hospitals, the stitches weakened from contact with body fluids and gave way while the patient was in transit. But as soon as the failing was discovered, instructions were sent forward substituting new procedures for the faulty methods.

The greatest credit is given by the Russians to the air ambulance service which brought in sixty-five per cent of all the patients. Since wounds of the chest are, more than almost any others, emergency wounds, the speed of transport and the comfort of the patient during transport play a vital part in lowering death rates. Linberg found that patients who had been moved by air were invariably in a better condition than those who had traveled by other means, even when comparable cases with an equal time-lag between wounding and reception at the hospital were considered. Since his hospital accepted cases from an entire army corps, patients were received at any time between the second and twentieth day after injury. The majority, thanks to plane transport, came in on the second or third day, directly from front line stations.

The Russian experience should serve to lay at rest the fears of American surgeons regarding air transport of patients suffering from chest wounds. These fears arose from the recognition of the fact that a patient with pneumothorax carries what amounts to a closed container of gas within the chest; this gas being air under ground-level pressure. When the plane reaches the rarefied atmosphere necessary for safe flight, this cache of air in the chest cavity tends to expand. At a little over fifteen thousand feet, it would normally double in volume. Thus a condition similar to pressure pneumothorax would set in, with the air inside the chest wall forcing the central wall over and compressing the other lung and the heart.

The Russian procedure did not solve this problem; it simply avoided it. The ambulance planes were equipped with pressure cabins, so that no matter how high the plane flew and how rarefied the outside air, the atmosphere within the cabin remained at ground pressures. Undoubtedly similar planes will be made available for any similar American evacuation project.

It should be noted that the Russian techniques differ but little, if at all, from those followed by present-day American and British surgeons. They differ from those of the latter part of World War I, the previous high mark in the surgery of war wounds of the chest, mainly in their emphasis on early treatment. The doctors of 1917 worked a revolution simply by cutting down on their reliance on natural healing and replacing this with planned surgical intervention. In fact, by insisting on early intervention in the case of open pneumothorax wounds, the death rate in World War I, for this particular type of wound, was cut from nearly ninety per cent to thirty per cent and less.

The doctors of today carry this change a step further and not only intervene but do so at the earliest possible moment. Emergency intervention in the field, such as the closing of an open chest wound, saves many men who would otherwise never reach a hospital at all. High-speed evacuation and the services of specialists in chest surgery save many more. The end result reflects itself in such figures as the three per cent death rate of the Linberg experiment.

Chest wounds are—or were—among the most deadly of battle injuries. But two classes of wounds, those of the spine and those of the abdomen, have always proved even more fatal. If we cannot, as in the case of chest wounds, report so dramatic a lowering of the death rate for these latter classes, we can still find much encouragement in the effect modern methods of field medicine and surgery have had on even these, the worst of war wounds.

Major Douglas Jolly, a volunteer surgeon in the Spanish Republican Army and author of that bible of all modern military surgeons, *Field Medicine in Total War*, has supplied the following list of factors influencing the prognosis (the doctors' word describing the patient's chances) for wounds of the abdomen:

(a) Site and direction of the wound.
(b) Organ or organs affected.
(c) Type of projectile.
(d) Physical condition of the wounded man at time of injury.
(e) Condition under which the operation takes place.
(f) Possibilities for blood transfusion.
(g) Time-lag between injury and operation.

When we examine this list, line by line, we find that in respect to two of these criteria, our soldiers today are neither better off nor worse off than those of 1918. Missiles that hit the abdomen will still hit from all directions and will still affect the various organs with approximately the same frequency. Under some circumstances, such as aerial strafing, abdominal wounds may more frequently be caused by bullets entering from the rear, but it is too early to say whether such wounds, as a group, would prove better or worse in prognosis than those incurred from the more traditional ground fighting.

In respect to the type of projectile the injuries of modern war may prove more severe. High-speed explosive shells and bombs send small, whirling fragments flying in all directions. These may cause an extremely small wound of entry yet bring on great damage within the body in their twisting flight.

Granting these passive or negative factors, we must still find that the balance lies in favor of the present-day soldier. Certainly among American troops, every measurement serves to indicate that the average soldier's physical condition today is better than that of his 1918 predecessor. Unless a very hard and very long war should badly lower this average, the men of the present army will have a decided advantage on this point. The conditions under which operations take place have likewise improved. While in exceptional circumstances, as was the case on Bataan Peninsula, these conditions will be fully as bad and even worse than anything met in France in 1918, on the average we have every right to expect them to be far better. This is true both because surgical equipment has been substantially improved in the last twenty-five years and because the motorization of transport and the development of mobile hospital units permit the present-day medical corps a far greater control of operative conditions than was ever before possible.

There remain Jolly's last two criteria, and for these tremendous advances have occurred since the last war. Where once the possibilities of blood transfusion were sharply limited, today almost every injured man can count on a dried-plasma or preserved-blood injection. Certainly no severely wounded abdominal case, except in the most tragic and exceptional of circumstances, will ever again fail of recovery for lack of a transfusion.

As for the time-lag factor, every new development in field surgery has served either to cut the lag between wounding and operation or to extend the patient's ability to endure the lag. Sir Cuthbert Wallace once analyzed a series of nearly six hundred abdominal cases of World War I, recording the number of deaths and recoveries according to the lapse of time before the wounded reached the operating table. Each passing hour served to raise the number of fatalities and to lower the chances of the wounded for survival, particularly each hour after the sixth. Today, such experiences as those of the Russians and of our own troops wherever they have fought, serve to indicate that most of the wounded, and certainly far more than ever before, can now be placed in the surgeon's hands before the six-hour period passes.[1] The use of the sulfa drugs, to delay the spread of infection, will serve further to buffer the chances of the abdominally wounded, for the greatest adverse factor after the six-hour period lies in the spread of infection. The sulfa drugs, by arresting this spread, help to extend the golden period by the few hours that may spell all the difference between life and death.

Wounds of the chest, abdomen, and spine still remain among wars' worst wounds. No single miracle has arisen which can wipe out their severity. Yet the combination of a series of advances in field medicine and in surgery is making for a radical reduction in death rates and recovery time. This, more than anything else, is the important and encouraging factor in the Linberg experiment. For though we cannot, as yet, count upon so satisfactory a reduction in mortality being obtained at all times and in all actions, we know that the Russians had no cards up their sleeves. What they did in the Russo-Finnish War is being duplicated today—with some important improvements no doubt— by every Allied medical service, Russian, British, American, and Chinese. And though we must still recognize the severity of these wounds, we must not lose sight of the fact that they constitute but a small fraction of all the wounds of war. Just how small a

[1] A more detailed description of how this is accomplished will be found in Chapter XIII.

fraction they are is demonstrated by the statistics for hospital admission for battle injuries of the A.E.F. in the last war, when out of 174,296 cases, these three groups combined accounted for less than five per cent of the total.

The individual soldier's chance of receiving any wound at all varies with the severity and duration of the war. In World War I, about ten per cent of all the American troops abroad, less than one half of one per cent, were hospitalized for wounds of the chest, spine, or abdomen. Only two in each thousand wounded succumbed to these wounds. This time we know already, the toll of wars' worst wounds will be proportionately less. How much less, only time can tell.

Chapter X

THE SULFA QUINTET

SEVEN years ago when our knowledge of sulfa was at a stage comparable to Wilbur Wright's first plane, we all marveled at the miracle of these pills that cured —actually *cured*—diseases which we had never been able to conquer before. The fact that we didn't know what made the drug work, nor how it worked nor even when it worked . . . that just made it so much the more marvelous. Today, when the real miracles of chemotherapy are just beginning to be unveiled, the story of the sulfa drugs is so much "old stuff" to most of us. A new addition to the sulfa family gets hardly any more notice than another Atlantic crossing.

The sulfa quintet may nonetheless prove more important toward winning the war than even the great ferry-plane services. For the diseases and deaths of warfare arise, in greatest number, precisely from the infectious agents the sulfa drugs are best able to fight and defeat. The sulfa family, already so important in peacetime, is proving decisive now in preventing and limiting epidemics, in arresting the spread of wound infections, in speeding up the process of recovery from everything from pneumonia to gonorrhea, from arthritis to dysentery.

The military importance of the sulfa drugs may, in fact, be measured with a fairly high degree of accuracy. Let's try it, in a rough way, for just one disease, pneumonia. We know that in the last war there were 45,774 hospitalized cases of pneumonia among United States troops. We know that 10,145 of these cases resulted in death, a death rate of slightly more than twenty-two per cent. We know that 1,845,758 days were lost by men sick with this single disease, with probably an equal number of days spent by other valuable personnel, such as doctors, nurses, ambulance drivers, cooks, etc. Each man was lost to service for an average of forty days.

Now let's look at some effects of sulfa therapy on civilian pneumonia rates. First we have to consider the matter of the incidence of pneumonia, for this is a disease that blossoms especially when the body has been weakened by some other infection, such as influenza. Against many of these infections which ultimately result in pneumonia, doctors now use one or another of the sulfa drugs. More patients survive the original disease without getting pneumonia at all, either because the sulfa drug cured the first disease handily or because it defeated the pneumococcus before the symptoms of pneumonia became clearly established.

Secondly, taking the people who actually do get pneumonia, we find that the death rate has been cut from somewhere in the range between twenty and thirty per cent to an average of around seven per cent. All of these figures vary, from year to year, with the type of pneumonia, with the age of the patients and with many another factor. Yet, over any large series of cases, like the nearly 25,000 studied by Dr. Maurice A. Schnitker, the drop in the death rate has run between sixty and seventy-five per cent. Only one-quarter to one-third as many deaths occur per hundred cases as did before the advent of the sulfa drugs. Even more important is the drop among younger patients, for the Army is made up of young men. Among patients under forty the mortality from pneumonia now runs about three and one-half per cent.

Finally, we must take the factor of duration of illness into consideration. With the sulfa drugs, the temperature is usually reduced to normal or nearly normal within seventy-two hours. It is not at all unusual for a pneumonia patient to return to his occupation within a week. Ten days seems to be the average time of hospitalization. This may still be on the high side, for an increasing number of the lighter cases are no longer sent into hospitals at all.

If we apply these figures to the Army in the last war,

we get the following results. First, the number of pneumonia cases must be cut by anywhere from ten to sixty per cent. We know that the incidence of pneumonia in our Army in 1941, a peacetime year, was less than half that of 1917, a comparable year of training rather than fighting. If we take this figure, we must cut our admissions to hospital for pneumonia by fifty per cent. But let us be conservative and figure that in wartime they might run somewhat higher. Nonetheless, every factor would still indicate a reduction in the number of cases from 45,774 to about 30,000 if today's conditions had prevailed in 1918.

Next we must consider the reduction in death rates. Again let us reject the extremely favorable figures of 1941, when the death rate in our Army was less than one-twentieth that of 1917. Let us instead take the average death rate among people under forty, three and one-half per cent. Applied to our thirty thousand cases, we would get an indicated death total of 1,050, about one-tenth of the actual figure for our Army in the last war. If we are even more conservative, and use the higher figures that now apply to the entire population, we get an indicated pneumonia death total of about 2,500, still only one-quarter of what it actually was in 1918.

Finally, we must consider the matter of days lost in the hospital. If we take ten days as an average and apply it to our figure of thirty thousand cases, we get three hundred thousand lost days, only one-sixth as many as before. If our thirty thousand pneumonia victims each gain this average month of recovery time, the army gains the equivalent of the services of two entire divisions for a month.

The armed forces actually make such calculations, not only for pneumonia, but for all diseases and injuries. For it is only by anticipating the hospital load that they can know how much equipment to build and ship, how many doctors and nurses and other help to train and transport to the zone of action. Naturally the Army's method of calculation is far more detailed than that which we have just used. The results, without question, are far more accurate as a basis for prediction. But that the sulfa drugs play a vital part in our war effort is apparent no matter what the method of calculation may be. For sulfa has cut the number of patients, cut the length of their stay, cut the development of complications, and cut the death rate all along the line.

Often the effect of the sulfa drugs proves even more startling than in the case of pneumonia. Gonorrhea has always been a scourge of armies, though perhaps slightly less so to American forces than to those of some other nations. The effect of this venereal disease is seldom reflected in mortality statistics; gonorrhea victims usually live to pass on their infection. But as a crippler of military personnel, the infection has no equal. In World War I, more than a quarter of a million men had to be hospitalized for a total loss of nearly four million days because of this single disease. The average stay in the hospital was sixteen days.

Then, in 1937, the first attempts were made to use sulfanilamide as a cure for gonorrhea. The results were so much better than anything attainable before that doctors everywhere made sulfanilamide their first choice for gonorrhea treatment. Yet quick cures were accomplished in only about half the cases and the nausea, and other toxic effects of the drug, made victims of the disease extremely reluctant to report their malady. They feared the cure more than the fever. In 1940 sulfapyridine replaced sulfanilamide for the treatment of gonorrhea. The cure rate went up to about ninety per cent, reactions dropped off, but still the doctors weren't quite satisfied. Within a year, they tried sulfathiazole and raised their rate of cure to ninety-five per cent. Most important of all, ninety per cent of the cases were cured within five days.

But very recently, even sulfathiazole is being dropped in favor of a fourth sulfa drug, the newer sulfadiazine. One of the many experiments with the drug was conducted by Captain Robert F. Parsons of the U. S. Navy Medical Corps. Captain Parsons used a series of thirty cases for test purposes and it is significant to note that he found it so difficult to get thirty cases for treatment that he had to shift his base of operations in the middle of his test. After collecting twenty patients at the Washington Naval Hospital he found his last ten cases, to complete the series, at the Portsmouth, New Hampshire, Naval Hospital. Yet despite this testimony to the effectiveness of the earlier sulfa drugs, the Navy wasn't satisfied. It wanted a hundred per cent cure and Captain Parsons was expected to find it if it could be found.

Of the thirty cases, not a single one offered any complaint nor showed any signs of a toxic reaction. Many of them volunteered the information that they were not aware of the slightest feeling of taking any drug. But for the requirements of the experiment each could have remained at his ordinary work. For that matter, all of them shortly returned to their stations, a one hundred per cent cure being achieved within ten days from the start of treatment. All except four of the men were cured within five days. Compared with the millions of days lost only a few years ago, this may seem just about perfect. But the Navy isn't quite satisfied, even yet. They don't like the fact that some cases still take "so long" to cure. Before the war is over, they expect to be able to reduce the treatment of gonorrhea to a matter of such routine nature that no man will ever be incapacitated by the disease and none will get the opportunity to pass on the infection.

Unlike gonorrhea, meningitis is one of the rarer military maladies. In the last war, some 4,831 cases were recorded among American troops. For two reasons, it has always been most feared by those entrusted with maintaining the health of fighting men. First, it is— or was—among the most deadly of diseases. Of our less than four thousand, 1918 cases, nearly forty per cent, died. Secondly, one form at least is violently infectious and there is always the danger that it may sweep through an army cantonment with devastating results.

The old military statistics on meningitis are deceptive, for they class as a single disease any infection of the meninges, the membranes enveloping the brain and spinal cord. Today meningitis is classified, according to the bacteria which bring it on, as streptococcal meningitis, pneumococcal meningitis, and meningococcal meningitis. This last disease is also known as cerebro-spinal fever. The death rate from it once ran as high as seventy and even ninety per cent. About 1906, immune sera, derived from the few patients who had recovered from earlier attacks, began to be used. Much credit was given to it for subsequent reductions in the death rate, particularly in the British Navy where the rate was cut from 61 per cent in 1915 to 32 per cent in the latter years of the first World War. Later comparisons with results achieved by other means in the British Army and among civil cases cast doubt upon the effectiveness of serum, although most authorities do credit it with some reduction of the death rate. It was not, however, until the sulfa drugs became available that any real victory could be chalked up. When Great Britain entered the war in 1939, the army medical authorities made ready for the usual winter epidemic of cerebro-spinal fever. If anything they knew that it might be more severe that first winter when men from all sections of the country, with varying degrees of natural or acquired immunity, would be crowded together in camps and barracks as easy marks for carriers who transmit the infection.

The epidemic came, as expected, in the early months of 1940, the most extensive epidemic ever recorded on the British Isles. But the doctors were ready. For three years, prior to that time, men such as H. S. Banks had been using sulfanilamide on the occasional, sporadic cases of the disease. They had had most encouraging results, with a death rate of only six per cent. Of course, they knew that between epidemics the virulence of the disease was low. Yet when the epidemic came, the sulfa drugs cut the death rate to the lowest figures ever achieved. Among civilians, only part of whom were treated by chemotherapy, the rate fell to less than twenty-four per cent. In the army, where the use of sulfanilamide under controlled conditions was the rule, the rate stood at exactly half that figure. Thus any question of the epidemic being a mild one was eliminated. It was proved, once and for all, that the sulfa drugs were the best method yet found for fighting this most deadly of bacterial diseases.

Individual reports showed even more favorable results. Dr. Banks had only twelve deaths in 120 cases. Dr. R. W. Cushing reported an army series of 124 cases with only 3.2 per cent fatality. Other forms of meningitis have likewise been made far less deadly by the sulfa family. Meninges infections caused by hemolytic streptococci, the bacteria that infects most wounds, once resulted in death for between ninety-five and one hundred per cent of all cases. Today the rate has been reduced to less than twenty per cent. Moreover, the incidence of the disease has been greatly cut, for sulfa treatment often prevents the spread of hemolytic infections which would eventually reach and penetrate the spinal canal or the brain.

An accurate evaluation of the all-over effect of the sulfa drugs on disease in the armed forces is extremely difficult if not impossible to work out. Not only have the methods of classifying diseases changed, making comparison difficult, but the diseases themselves change with time. Many are cyclic in their virulence, so that the figures for any two years are not strictly comparable. The general health of the troops, their average age, the conditions under which they fight and a host of other factors affect the picture. Yet, as we did with pneumonia, a rough comparison may be made and may prove useful, provided we do not forget its limitations.

In the twenty months of our participation in the last war, over three and a half million men were hospitalized for diseases of one sort or another. Since the army totaled only a little over four million, it is clear that many men were sent to hospitals more than once. More than fifty-seven thousand of these men died. The average stay in the hospitals was eighteen days and the total number of days lost reached the astronomical figure of 62,681,428.

At least thirty of the diseases for which these men were hospitalized are susceptible to treatment with the sulfa drugs. These account for nearly one-quarter of all the days lost and for a somewhat larger portion of the deaths. If recovery rates such as are being experienced in civil practice today could have applied to these cases, the death rate for this group could have been cut to between one-quarter and one-half of what it actually was. The time loss could certainly have been halved.

The treatment of disease as distinguished from battle injuries is but one phase—and not the most important one—of sulfa's war work. Of far more importance is the manner in which the sulfa drugs are used to fight infection in war wounds. At many another point in this volume we have referred to the use of these drugs, in fighting burn infections, in combination with plaster casts in the Trueta-Orr fracture treatment, in treating chest, abdominal, and brain wounds and in reconstructive surgery. The over-all picture is best portrayed in a calculation of the British author, F. Sherwood Taylor. During the first World War, Mr. Taylor notes, some seven and a quarter million deaths occurred (among all the warring nations) due to injuries as distinguished from deaths due to illness. Three-quarters took place on the battlefield. Many of these latter can be avoided nowadays, and sulfa plays no small part in that victory.

But one-quarter of all wound deaths occurred among patients who had reached a hospital. The chief cause of these hospital deaths (still according to Mr. Taylor) was not the wounds themselves. It was a single, pervasive form of bacteria, the hemolytic streptococcus. Colonel Leonard Colebrook, one of the great living authorities on this particular bug, ascribes to the hemolytic streptococcus eighty to ninety per cent of all war wound deaths.

For generations doctors have known about this germ. But they knew of only a few ways of fighting it, none of them any too effective. The best way was also the simplest: sanitation and antisepsis. This they had proved in the fight against childbed fever caused by the wound-loving hemolytic bug. The doctors had learned to a degree how to prevent the bug from getting into contact with the woman's organs, lacerated and "wounded" by the labor of childbirth. They set up special maternity wards, sterilized their hands and clothes before entering delivery rooms, used separate nursing staffs isolated from the general run of patients. Instead of losing one mother in thirty, as had been the case around 1870, they had cut the rate of infection until, in 1935, in England, only one such death occurred for six hundred and fifty births.

Many doctors were satisfied. The death-rate reduction looked good, on the record. But among those who did not like the picture was Leonard Colebrook, who was then serving as a surgeon at Queen Charlotte's Maternity Hospital in London. Colebrook knew that his hospital had been losing, through death, one-quarter of all the women who had caught the infection despite all their doctors' precautions. As soon as the discovery of the first sulfa drug was announced in 1935, he started to use it on every puerperal sepsis case, sixty-four in all in 1935 and 1936. Instead of the expected sixteen deaths, only three occurred. The death rate had been cut to less than one-fifth. Later workers have had even better experiences. Present rates run as low as 1.4 per cent.

Puerperal sepsis is hardly a disease of warfare. But it differs by only a very little from any other wound infection. The hemolytic streptococcus is not very discriminating; it will invade any wound if it gets a chance. And it usually does get its chance, particularly in warfare when the difficulty of maintaining antisepsis is many times multiplied. If it gains access to a wound and causes a local infection, it may bring on severe fever and swelling. The doctors call this *cellulitis*. If it invades the tissues and passes into the blood stream, it causes *streptococcal septicemia* or blood poisoning. If it gains access to the deeper layers of the skin, it may spread along the underskin, causing *erysipelas*. It may invade the ear. And it may get to the brain, causing *streptococcal meningitis*.

Before the advent of the sulfa drugs, there was very little that the doctors could do about these wound infections, as the death rates well indicate. They could attempt to keep the germ from reaching the wound; but they knew in advance that the attempt would be a losing one all too often. If the man didn't enter the hospital with the germ already in his wound, he usually picked it up very shortly from a neighbor, a nurse, or any other contact. Attempts at prevention, that centered around keeping the wound clean or antiseptic, also failed in a high percentage of all cases. Once infection occurred, the best you could hope for was a long-delayed recovery. Frequently the amputation of a limb was the only way of saving life, often even that couldn't help.

But with the sulfa drugs, medicine had something that could fight the infection no matter where it seated itself. Doctors began to give the drug by mouth to every patient entering a military hospital, whether infection had shown itself or not. The death rate dropped dramatically. Then they started to give the drug in the advance dressing stations. The number of contaminated wounds that matured into infections dropped still further. Men who once would have reached a hospital in a hopeless condition, now were brought in, even forty-eight hours after injury, capable of full and speedy recovery. Finally, they decided to give each soldier his own supply of sulfanilamide so that he could begin taking the life-saving drug as soon as he was hit. Where surgery could not possibly move up to the front lines, chemotherapy could and did. It arrested the development of streptococcal infections and by doing so gave surgery a chance on the very cases which once died before or despite surgical treatment.

Yet the sulfa drugs had their limitations. For like any drug, they had their therapeutic range. The function of a drug is to attack the invading organism, either to kill it outright or help the body in the killing. But drugs which kill germs also kill human cells. Were this not so, we would have utterly defeated bacterial diseases long ago, for we have many antiseptic drugs that can instantly kill almost any bacteria. The drugs we can use, however, are those with a favorable therapeutic range—those which are less deadly to man than to the invading germ.

With the sulfa drugs, the range is favorable. Most people, but not all people, can take enough of the drug by mouth to establish a high enough blood concentration to defeat an invasion in some remote part of the body. But, if you take too much of the drug—say, enough to defeat some particularly virulent infection—you will be poisoned by the very chemical that is supposed to save you. Reactions will set in, to use the polite terminology by which doctors avoid the dread word—poisoning.

The first approach which scientists took towards this problem of the sulfa drugs was to seek some less toxic variation of sulfanilamide, a drug that would either be more powerful against germs or less powerful against man. That is how the sulfa family grew. Sulfanilamide was replaced, for certain diseases, by sulfapyridine. This was particularly more powerful against pneumonia and gonorrhea bacteria. At first it was thought to be less toxic than sulfanilamide, but later checks on several long series of cases showed the toxicity to be about equal. Since, however, it was more effective against certain diseases, you could either use smaller doses—and thus avoid the toxicity problem—or you could lick the disease so quickly that the drug could be discontinued before the patient suffered any really dangerous toxic reactions.

The next drug in the quintet was sulfathiazole. This was more rapidly absorbed into the blood stream and therefore it acted more quickly. It was equally effective for most diseases, and, most important of all, it was far less toxic. Against staphylococcal infections, it was much more effective than its two predecessors. Thus for many diseases, sulfathiazole replaced the earlier drugs. For others, sulfanilamide and sulfapyridine are still used.

Sulfadiazine was next in line, coming into experimental use in the fall of 1940 and into general use only very recently. It is definitely less toxic than any of the others. At first it was thought to be as good but no better than the other drugs, but more recent work indicates that it has the dual advantage of doing a better job against disease while endangering the patient far less.

The last drug in the quintet is a specialist. Sulfaguanidine was planned even before it was discovered. The other four drugs weren't too effective against diseases of the intestinal tract simply because they were so largely absorbed into the blood stream. Working on this problem at Johns Hopkins Hospital, Dr. Marshall and a group of associates sought a sulfa drug that would be poorly absorbed from the intestine. They found it in sulfaguanidine, a drug that develops from fifty to two hundred and fifty times higher concentration within the intestine than it does in the blood. The difference is exactly that between buckshot and a bullet. If you are trying to get at a general infection, say an infection of the blood stream, you use buckshot and bring the bacterial-birds down wherever they are on the wing. But if you want to get one particular infection which is localized in the intestinal tract, you use the sulfaguanidine bullets and you know that your shots will strike home.

The principal use for sulfaguanidine is in the treatment of bacillary dysentery, a disease particularly common in military life. The drug, properly administered, is virtually non-toxic. It clears up most cases in from three to five days, without hospitalization. It will probably also be of use in fighting cholera and the early stages of typhoid fever, should these prove to be a problem. Such cases it is hoped will be few indeed among American troops in view of the compulsory typhoid inoculations which every American soldier undergoes and in view of the sanitary standards maintained by the Army.

Paralleling the search for less toxic, more potent variants of the sulfa drugs, there has been another development of major military importance. It came about through a different approach to the same old problem, namely, making the drug more effective against germs and less toxic to man.

Doctors, particularly those who did not thoroughly understand the problems of chemotherapy, were prone in the early days to increase the dosage of the drug for desperate cases. They saw the normal or recommended dose failing to defeat the invading germs. They took a chance, increasing the dose in the hope of gaining a sufficient blood concentration to defeat the bacteria. Sometimes they and their patients were lucky and despite severe reactions, the drug killed the bugs before it killed the patient. When they failed and their patients died, the doctors could comfort themselves with the thought that anything else, any other procedure, would also have ended in death. At least, they had tried.

But others, particularly the military men, sought some better method. It seemed silly to them to have to dose the entire body in order to establish a germ-fighting concentration of the drugs at the site of infection. Wrestling with this headache, these surgeons and their friends, the bacteriologists, began to think of a new way to use the sulfa drugs. They said to themselves, "Suppose we were to put the drug directly onto the wounded area? What then? Can we not establish a high enough concentration at the point where concentration counts? At the same time, won't we protect our patient against the dangers inherent in overdosing the whole body with sulfa drugs?"

The idea was a natural one and presented extremely inviting prospects. But other doctors equally prominent sounded a dire note of warning. As late as 1940, Dr. W. B. Thrower, consulting physician to the major British producer of the sulfa drugs, May and Baker

Ltd., inveighed against the idea of local application. He said that the drugs might act like foreign bodies if placed in the wound, that they might affect the nervous system, that application by mouth might give sufficiently high concentrations while application directly into the wound might be ineffective.

Dr. Thrower had every theoretical reason for propounding these views. As far as theory was concerned, he was right and the young iconoclasts were dead wrong. Luckily, the physicians actually in the field, the doctors who worked at Dunkirk and in Libya and the general practitioners who fought the London and Coventry blitzes, had their own ideas and chose to follow them. Perhaps it was because if they failed no one, least of all their poor patients, would be worse off. If they succeeded, then once again practice would have run ahead of theory and the theorists would have to beat an orderly retreat and announce new theories on the basis of "newly discovered evidence." There would be no hard feeling on either side, just hard work.

So in spite of the eminent Dr. Thrower and many another, the method of local implantation of sulfa onto wounds became more and more popular. By 1941, no one questioned the efficacy of the procedure. A Dr. Hawkins was able to show that, against the weight of predictions, the drug was absorbed, usually within twenty-four hours. After that, it was no longer present as crystals which could be considered as dangerous foreign bodies. Colonel Colebrook applied sulfanilamide powder to sixty-two wounds infected with hemolytic streptococci and the organisms were cleared out in from three to four days. In America, Key and Burford ran a controlled experiment. They had ninety-four cases of compound fractures in series before the use of local implantations. Twenty-five of these developed infections. Seven had gas gangrene and five amputations were necessary. Then they used local applications on forty compound fractures, quite as severe as the first series. Only two cases, or five per cent, developed any infection. No gangrene. No amputations.

After that, it was simply a matter of learning more about the best methods of local application. The doctors began to use the powders, particularly sulfanilamide, on all sorts of wounds. They tried using it on brain wounds and it worked. They tried it on abdominal wounds and it worked. They began to use it even when the wound was one of their own making, on appendicitis cases. And still it worked. They used it on burns, in the Pickrell sulfadiazine spray, and found it effective. They used it under skin transplants and again it was effective. By July, 1941, the Navy specified sulfanilamide powder for the battle bags of hospital corpsmen. Local application had become a standardized, fully recognized procedure. At Pearl Harbor, local application had its ultimate test. According to every report, the drug came through even better than its most hopeful proponents had expected. Captain W. H. Michael of the Navy Medical Corps reported that *there never has been a group of war wounds as free of infection* as those in Hawaii.

Captain George A. Eckert of the Navy pointed out an unlooked-for advantage when he reported the deliberate delaying of treatment in cases of shock. During the first World War it was considered that the sooner a gunshot or shrapnel wound was cleaned and débrided, the less chance there would be of infection. But that meant taking chances with shock. The added strain of surgery sometimes killed men who were operated upon while still under the initial influence of their wounds. There was little the doctors could do about it; if they wished to avoid the danger of infection they must, perforce, place their patients under the danger of early surgery.

But at Pearl Harbor another procedure was followed. After two unexpected deaths under early surgery, the Navy doctors changed their routine. They operated no more on patients with shrapnel wounds until recovery from shock had taken place. During the intervening several days, the wounds were left wide open, packed with sulfanilamide powder and covered with sterile dressings. In only one case out of twenty-five did infection make headway. The new procedure cannot of course be used in all instances. In abdominal wounds, in hemorrhage cases, or when the shrapnel is in contact with important structures, early surgical intervention is essential. But for the rest, sulfanilamide powder used liberally in shrapnel wounds enables the present-day military surgeon to deliberately defer surgery until the patient becomes readjusted and the risk of operation is minimized.

Thus today the sulfa drugs stand as our greatest single weapons against both disease and wound infections. Throughout the world they are saving lives daily, cutting down recovery time, eliminating even the need for entering a hospital in many cases. They bring solace and a sense of security to the wounded. They permit the physician to plan his treatment, the surgeon to plan his operation with less worry about the need for speed and hurry. They save minds and limbs and looks . . . and still we have not begun to reach the end of the sulfa miracle.

For today we have only a quintet of sulfa drugs, the forerunners without any doubt of other, more effective, speedier, less toxic, and more powerful sulfa compounds. Half a dozen such are in experimental use right now. More than that, we have the beginning of an understanding of how the sulfa drugs work. For strange as it may seem, all the amazing progress we have made in the last seven or eight years has been made in semi-darkness. We knew the drugs did certain things under certain conditions, but we knew very little of the *How* and practically nothing of the *Why* about these performances.

But step by step, medical theorists—who are of much more use than it may have seemed a few pages back— have moved towards a working explanation of the mode of action of these drugs. Today there are at least five major theories and any number of variants.[1] These hypotheses all answer some of our questions and thus contain some truth. None, as yet, explains every phe · nomenon of the sulfa drugs but that does not mean that they are not useful. For in science, any hypothesis is useful if it helps to guide our further investigations along productive lines. The value of such theories in advancing our knowledge and use of these drugs and in leading us towards other effective drugs is demonstrated by a single development arising from the Para-aminobenzoic Acid Theory of Stamp and Woods. This theory postulates that para-aminobenzoic acid, a substance very similar to sulfanilamide, is the food on which bacteria grow. Sulfanilamide competes with para-aminobenzoic acid, interfering with the bacteria's

---

[1] These theories, dealing as they do with the vastly complicated subject of bacterial metabolism, are themselves complex and can be explained only in chemical and metabolic concepts unfamiliar to all but the trained technician. Let me be frank to say that I do not understand them myself, though Heaven knows, I've tried. Readers who wish to pursue them may find the treatment contained in Dr. M. A. Schnitker's work, *Sulfanilamide Compounds in the Treatment of Infections,* an exceedingly lucid introduction.

use of this substance. On the other hand, if enough para-aminobenzoic acid is present, the sulfa drug is inhibited in *its* action. All this was suggested before the recent identification of para-aminobenzoic acid as one of the vitamins of the B-complex. When it did pop up in the unraveling of the B-vitamin structure, the theory of Woods suggested that doctors look into the advisability of forbidding the administration of B-vitamin when a patient is taking a course of sulfa drugs. Today this question, which otherwise could not even have been posed, is being studied. If the Woods theory is correct, medicine has learned how to avoid a dangerous combination of vitamin and drug. On the other hand, further studies may lead to the demolition or change of the Woods theory, if it should prove that taking B-vitamins and Sulfa at the same time has no ill effect.

A similar by-product of the Para-aminobenzoic Acid Theory cautions physicians against using certain local anaesthetics, derived from the acid, simultaneously with the sulfa drugs. Here the tests of investigators seem to already confirm the Woods theory, for such anaesthetics definitely inhibit the action of sulfapyridine.

The importance of all these theories, in so far as the war is concerned, is that they indicate that sulfa progress has by no means reached a dead end. Before the war is over, the military doctors will have contributed much to the hoard of clinical knowledge against which all theories must check. The laboratory technicians, who seem to be sitting in splendid isolation away from the war, may in turn be responsible for the explanation of sulfa action which will make today's performance look like witchcraft against the cures the sulfa family will work tomorrow.

Chapter XI

THE NEW MAGIC OF LOCAL ANAESTHESIA

IN 1937, the officers of the Japanese Kwantung Army were feeling their oats. They had conquered Manchuria, walked over the northern provinces of China, and were ready, at last, to tackle the Russian Bear. If the cautious and timorous politicians of Tokio doubted their readiness, they proposed to prove it to them and to the world by invading Outer Mongolia, that little known region north of the Gobi Desert from which they could flank the entire Russian Far Eastern establishment.

For weeks they gathered their equipment, for even the brash young officers of Japan knew that the new Russian armies were not going to be as easy to overrun as had been the disorganized, ill-armed Manchurian forces. The Japanese jingoes were not ready for a full-fledged war, but they proposed to push the Russians around a little and to demonstrate to the home folks that a war with the Soviets might be a very profitable venture. So with banners flying, with tanks and trucks and armored cars, the little men of Nippon crossed the Mongolian border at Lake Hassan.

The battle was hidden well away from war correspondents and it was only weeks afterwards that the first detailed reports began to filter through from both sides. The Russians, it developed, were not caught napping. With planes and tanks they blasted the Japs out of their territory and back into Manchuria so fast that most of their equipment and thousands of men were left on the field. The Japanese called it an "incident," said "So sorry," and proceeded to march their men off in other directions where conquest seemed easier. But in point of numbers this was no mere border scrape. Thousands of men were engaged on both sides, the fighting went on for weeks and the Russians convinced the Japanese, once and for all, that the Bear had new claws and would fight.

On the Russian side, the battle served the major purpose of warding off, at relatively small cost, an all-out war. But it had its minor results, as well, and some of these in retrospect have proved of major importance because they helped prepare the Red Army for its great test. The moment the actual battle was over, military commissions began to investigate every detail of the action. Officers who had done well were promoted; those who had been backward in their efforts were shifted, sent back to school, or even reduced to the ranks. The tank plants of Moscow and Stalingrad and Magnitogorsk revised their designs to eliminate defects and profit by the lessons of the fight on the

Manchurian plains. Artillery was redesigned, plane plans revised, even new automatic, motorized bakeries were developed because bread had been slow in getting to the fighting men and stale when it got there.

Not the least of the overhauling jobs was concerned with the medical services. Throughout the Soviet Union doctors stood up and criticized, suggested, deplored, and discussed the shortcomings as well as the achievements of the medical branches. Some changes were made immediately. In other departments, the medical profession decided that vast new fields of research must be opened up, so that when Soviet forces fought again, new techniques would reduce the death rate and limit disabilities among the survivors. The process is one familiar to the American Army which has, likewise, converted hindsight into foresight after every one of our own wars.

One of the things that stirred up a storm of controversy was the matter of anaesthesia. To the layman, anaesthetics are just anaesthetics. If he distinguishes between them at all, he classifies them as "local" anaesthetics and thinks of the novocaine injection his dentist shoots into his gums before an extraction, or as "general" anaesthetics and thinks of the pulsating bag of the gas administration apparatus as he has seen it in a Lionel Barrymore movie. It would be wonderful for the medical student if the whole field of anaesthesia could be covered by these simple alternatives. But matters are by no means so simple. There are several score of different anaesthetics, each desirable under certain circumstances, each completely useless under other conditions, each affecting the patient in its own pet ways prior to, during, and after an operation. Thus, even in civil practice, the surgeon must consider his anaesthetics quite as carefully as any other phase of his operative procedure.

Under wartime operating conditions, however, the problem is further complicated. Certain of the general anaesthetics require elaborate equipment which is not easily portable and therefore unsuited to front-line work. Other anaesthetics are highly explosive. These must be rejected for use on naval vessels and wherever the danger of explosion is sufficient to call for caution. Even when explosive gases (such as cyclopropane) are used, great care must be exercised to isolate the operating theater from spark-making electrical equipment and from X-ray apparatus. Still other anaesthetics, which may be used with facility under most circumstances, are undesirable because of their after-effects. The nausea and possible retching of an etherized patient is hardly desirable when chest wounds or abdominal wounds are to be dealt with. Some anaesthetic agents are distinctly undesirable for patients suffering from shock. Others may be used only for certain regions of the body, being either completely impractical or less desirable than alternatives for other regions.

The Russians found themselves aligned into two general schools of thought. On the one hand, there were the majority of the army field doctors, who stood up for general anaesthetics. Admitting all the defects of the all-over anaesthetics, including the bulk of the equipment and the need for skilled anaesthetists, they still maintained that "generals" such as ether, nitrous-oxide-plus-oxygen, ethylene, and cyclopropane were more practicable than were the "local" drugs. To support their arguments they told how inconvenient it had been to use ampoules of procaine. They reported that the two per cent solutions of this drug which had been provided for them had proved to be highly toxic and had to be used in such small quantities that the patient was often incompletely anaesthetized and felt great pain during the operation. They said that their patients complained, and rightfully, about the pain caused by blunt and thick needles, when they tried to inject local drugs. In sum, they said, " 'Local' anaesthetics may be all right in theory but we, who have had to use them in the field, find that we can get better, quicker, and more thorough results by using a general anaesthetic." Having made this point, they proceeded to confuse their arguments by each standing up for some one particular drug. Some said "chloroform," others said "ether." Still others called for "chloro-ethyl," at least for short operations.

Against all these arguments, the proponents of local

anaesthetics tended to throw their own answers. "If needles were too thick," they said, "use smaller needles, thin ones with sharp points that wouldn't hurt." They pointed out that under ether the going-to-sleep process was slow, prolonging the time of the operation. They showed that other drugs were highly critical. Too little and the patient felt the pain, too much and you poisoned him with an overdose. They remarked upon the post-operative excitement caused by some of the general drugs, the dangers to shocked patients, and the complications arising when the supply of trained personnel for gas administration failed during action.

Amid all the shouting, carried on as medical arguments usually are in terms of serious articles, where the words, "I beg to differ" really imply that one's opponent is at least a numbskull and possibly worse—amidst all this, some doctors on the "local" team began to indulge in what the Russians call "self-criticism." Their reasoning summed up to the conclusion that what the "general" men were saying about local anaesthesia might be partially true. The thing to do was to improve the process of local anaesthesia to a point where the merits inherent in the local drugs would not, any longer, be counterbalanced by defects and where the advantages over general anaesthesia would be so obvious that all would adopt the best procedure. Here again, the Russian doctors resembled our own in their love for a free-for-all—a fight that ends in a synthesis of all arguments and all methods into some solution that is better than anyone who started the fight ever thought possible.

The man most responsible for the development of the new Russian technique of local anaesthesia is Professor A. V. Vishnevsky. In 1938, he tackled the problem with the idea that the theory of "local" anaesthesia was correct but that the application methods were primitive. To bring the methods up to the possibilities of his drugs, as he saw them, Vishnevsky devised what he called the "creeping infiltration method," a technique designed to be simple, speedy, and easy of application, even under war conditions. Instead of using one or two injections of his anaesthetic drug in concentrated form, Vishnevsky used large quantities of very dilute solutions of procaine. But he took advantage of anatomy and injected his solution between the various layers of tissue, into the anatomical pockets that surround muscles and internal organs. Thus, with speed, he placed his solution into contact with large areas of tissue, securing a rapid anaesthetization by the contact of the relatively weak drugs with all the local small nerves.

The method required some skill in its application but not any more than the average surgeon, qualified to cut the tissues he anaesthetizes, can be counted upon to possess. Vishnevsky's idea was that the doctor could be his own anaesthetist, since he would inject his drugs as he proceeded with his operation.

One of the important effects claimed for the system by its author was a minimization of post-operative shock. He cited figures of the American, George Washington Crile, on amputations during the last war to show that mortality fell off greatly whenever local drugs replaced general anaesthesia. Later, Vishnevsky was to make even more far-reaching claims for his procedure, but in 1938 he limited himself to the suggestion that it be tried out under war circumstance at the first opportunity.

Early in 1939, Dr. I. M. Synovich conducted a long series of experiments to determine just how dilute a solution could be used and just how great a quantity of fluid might be injected without harming the patient. Procaine, he found, could be used in dilutions of as little as one part in ten thousand of water. With so weak a solution, Synovich made the theoretical claim that as much as 25,000 cubic centimeters could be utilized in a single operation without harming the patient. He did not propose to use so great a quantity—six gallons, when translated into English measurements. But he cited the figure to show the great margin of safety the drug would possess. In actual operations, seldom more than a thousand cubic centimeters are utilized but this is enough to give complete anaesthesia over the injected region within only two minutes. The insensitivity to pain lasted from four to six hours.

Soon a whole school of surgeons sprang up who were using the creeping infiltration method on all sorts of cases and singing its praises at every Russian medical meeting. In Moscow, Dr. G. M. Novikov reported on a series of 3,180 emergency operations in ninety-eight per cent of which the new method was used. This group was a typical cross section of the Moscow population. They ranged in age from a tot of three to oldsters in their eighties. More than one-third of these were traumatic cases, civil-life wounds caused by auto or industrial accidents, falls, explosions, stabs, hunting accidents, and so forth.

Sixty-five cases came into the hospital with penetrating wounds of the abdomen. At Lake Hassan, such cases had shown a mortality of fifty-five per cent. Yet Novikov, using Vishnevsky's anaesthetic method and Vishnevsky's dilute anaesthetic solution, cut this rate to 36.8 per cent.

In one hundred and fifty-four cases in which major amputations were performed under local anaesthesia, the mortality at the Moscow hospital was only 14.7 per cent. At Lake Hassan the figure had stood at 18.7 per cent and the general mortality from amputations in the entire Ukraine that year reached 22.8 per cent.

Yet for all that, the deep infiltration method was still to win its spurs in war. Surgeons could argue, and did, that it was all very well to show figures of low mortality in civil practice, but war was different. "For one thing," they asked, "wouldn't the new method take longer? If the surgeon had to act as his own anaesthetist, wouldn't he fall behind in his work when the flow of casualties began to mount during an active period at the front?"

Then, early in 1940, the Soviet-Finnish War broke out. Vishnevsky and his associates got the chance they had been waiting for. They had made some pretty bold and brash claims by now. Either they would prove themselves right and establish their method once and for all or they might find themselves the laughing stock of their profession. A medical unit was formed, consisting of three surgeons, Vishnevsky, Protopopov, and Pshenichnikov, aided by a graduate nurse, Kosynkova. The unit journeyed up to Leningrad and waited for orders. Within a few days they found themselves pulling up a snow-packed road, through lanes of branchless tree stumps, past deep-gutted shell craters newly covered with snow. The tractor that drew their sled sputtered and coughed in the forty-degree below zero cold. Then it stopped altogether.

The driver pointed through the falling snow to a fast disappearing footpath. "You'll have to walk in the back way, comrades," he said, pointing, "only the evacuation ambulances use the main road."

"But are you sure we're there?" asked Kosynkova,

who like the rest could see nothing all about but burnt-
over forest.

"You're there, all right," said the tractorman, starting up his motor and reversing his caterpillars for a
turn. "It's about a hundred yards to your left."

They trudged through the knee-deep path, the sound
of the guns to the distant north making them feel all
the more lost. The ground rose a little and they
climbed the small ridge, perhaps ten feet high in all,
but, in that flat country, a ridge. Below them, stood a
single white-garbed guard. "Where's the hospital?"
they asked.

"*This* is the hospital," he answered, pointing behind
him to a large shell crater which, now that they looked
closely, did seem somewhat different from the others
they had passed. The snow drifted into all the craters,
but this one was fuller and pitched upwards towards
its center. The guard led them down a ramp and
brushed aside a white canvas curtain and they found
themselves standing in the vestibule of a tent. From
around the edges of an inner curtain a warm current
of air greeted them. Then the second canvas was drawn
aside and they met the surgeon-in-charge.

"Welcome to our hospital," he began. Then noting
the amazed look on their faces he continued, "No, this
isn't the hospital itself. That's in the next two craters.
This is the staff's sleeping tent. See, we've made room
for you already."

Then he began to conduct them through his hospital, proudly, like a young boy. He took them outside and they walked along a path to the main road. An ambulance drove up and a squad of soldiers threw a white tarpaulin over the entire car, forming a tunnel between its rear doors and the entrance to a reception tent. "You see, we protect our men against a chill," said the young surgeon. "These men are only two hours from the front. We seldom get a case that has been wounded more than ten hours before. Our ambulance service is working at good tempo. That means that secondary wound shock has seldom set in and we do everything we can to see that it doesn't get any encouragement."

Inside the tent he showed them his sorting procedure. Here another young surgeon, aided by two medical orderlies, separated the men and sent those in surgical need toward the operating tent. Others passed through a canvas curtain to the dressing section, where minor wounds were cleaned and bandaged.

Through the rear of the tent their guide conducted them past another sailcloth curtain and into a canvas tunnel. "We've connected five shell craters in all here with our tunnels. Our airmen have tried to spot this place but the camouflage is perfect. From the air, you would not know that there was anything here, let alone a hospital that treats upwards of five hundred serious cases a week." They now moved into the first of the classification tents. The light filtered through the canvas itself and through a few white glass windows set high in the tent walls. All around them nurses were busy providing the wounded with their preliminary surgical attention. In one corner they recognized the Red Army's standard blood-bank cabinets and saw a young sergeant being given a transfusion. At other tables they noticed the standard tetanus and gas gangrene prophylactic injection procedures.

But their faces fell when they entered the last tent. This was divided into two sections by a partition. On one side the final preparations were carried on prior to actual operation. Across the partition powerful dome lights shown down upon two operating tables. The eyes of all four visitors turned to the heads of both tables. There they fixed upon two complete sets of gas anaesthesis apparatus; tanks, pipes, masks, valves, dials and all. Pshenichnikov started to say something but Vishnevsky touched his arm and they passed in silence through a final canvas tunnel, finding themselves once again in the tent to which they had originally been brought.

Seated at last and with warm glasses of strong Russian tea held between their hands, the circle of doctors began to talk. Tactfully, Vishnevsky praised what he had seen; the organization was perfect, the layout a vast improvement over former practice, the attention given to the men was obviously of a high order. In fact, he had only one criticism.

The hospital chief and his assistants looked anxiously at the famous man who had come all the way from Moscow to honor their unit. "Yes, what criticism did the professor have?"

Then started a battle royal. On one side stood the practical men, the divisional surgeons who had worked as a team now, without ceasing, twenty-four hours round the clock for twenty-two days. They used general anaesthetics and they proposed to stand by them. They had tried local anaesthetics; they might be fine back in Moscow but you simply couldn't propose to use them up here at the front where every moment saved might save not only the life that lay on your table but the life that waited out beyond the canvas curtain and perhaps the ones beyond that. True, general anaesthetics sometimes led to post-operative complications. Granted, evacuation might be more dangerous when ether or gas was utilized. Admittedly, patients in a state of shock gained nothing; perhaps even lost ground, when under ether or gas. But for all that, the field surgeon had to watch out for the main chance. Time was the touchstone of success in military surgery and no method, no matter how ingenious, could win out if it took more time.

Vishnevsky and his fellow visitors listened to all this, though they had heard it before—many, many times before. The professor let the others argue, until every point had been covered and recovered. Then, between sips of tea, he explained, "We know your arguments, comrades. Maybe they're right and maybe they're wrong. That is exactly why I've come up here, because the time for arguments is over. You've got two operating tables in there. I propose to borrow one and we'll see which method produces the best results."

The resident chief looked around at his assistants. Someone shrugged his shoulders. Another shook his head with a motion that said neither "yes" nor "no." The silence grew as cold as the air outside. Finally, the hospital director said, "When will you want to start, Professor?"

"Right now," Vishnevsky answered and began to change into his operating clothes.

For the next ninety-six hours, the two teams ran a race. Each of the three visiting doctors worked for eight hours and slept or watched the rival team for the intervening four. There were always two surgeons at that second table. They had a time with the nurse, Kosynkova. She wouldn't take time out at all, until literally ordered to go to bed or back to Leningrad.

Soon everyone around the place, even the convalescent patients, knew what was going on. It was too serious a matter for the serious Russians to bet on, but there was no rule—moral or otherwise—against keeping score. The records clerk became the most popular woman in the hospital. Even the ambulance drivers, who never before bothered to enter the tents, now managed to find some excuse on each trip to go in and find out the score from her.

The only figures they could get the first day concerned actual operations performed. These showed little. For a few hours both teams ran neck and neck. Then the general anaesthesia team drew ahead for a while. Everybody said, "What did I tell you?" Soon, however, it was neck and neck again, and by the second morning, the visitors from Moscow had taken a definite, if small, lead. This they held until the test of methods had ended.

The doctors and the more serious-minded attendants did not of course reduce the experiment to the level of a team match. The realization was always present that these were human lives being counted. Speed was important, but speed alone was nothing. They watched, instead, how the difficult cases fared under each method. What they saw on the local anaesthesia side made their eyes open.

There was, for instance, Soldier N., brought in with a bullet wound which had penetrated his stomach sideways just above the navel. Both the entrance and exit wounds were badly lacerated, with raw, torn edges, because the bullet had struck a rib on the right side and gone out sideways. Placed under local anaesthesia, the primary incisions into the abdominal cavity were made only to disclose it flooded with blood. More of the anaesthetizing fluid was injected into the mesentery, the fold of tissue that encloses the intestine and connects it to the abdominal wall. From here the fluid filtered back into the back wall of the stomach, anaesthetizing the entire region. Then the doctors sutured the several wounds of the mesentery itself, sewed up four wounds of the intestine, closed the abdominal cavity, treated the wounds of the abdominal wall and thus completed the operation. The hands of the clock, to which all eyes turned as the soldier was carried off, had moved but thirty minutes.

Soldier N. would in any army have been considered a very serious case, with at best a fifty-fifty chance of survival. Yet his post-operative period passed smoothly, as if the man had had some minor flesh wound. Within four days he was in good enough condition to be transferred to an interior zone hospital, where he made a prompt, undramatic, and uneventful recovery.

Another case was that of Soldier L., as the Russians like to tag their case histories. This man had been caught in a shrapnel burst and suffered injuries of the skull, chest, stomach, right shoulder, and right leg. A gaping wound in the chest hissed with every breath, as the air pressure of his lungs escaped through the hole. The man had lost much blood and was in an advanced state of shock when brought in, so advanced in fact that general anaesthesia would almost certainly have brought death on the operating table. Yet under creeping infiltration local anaesthesia, the hole in the chest was closed and sealed. Then the abdomen was opened and seven wounds of the small intestine sutured. Next the doctors turned to the skull, removed the fractured bone, cleared up the brain damage and closed the wound.

On the fourth day, Soldier L. was removed from the field hospital. It is very doubtful whether a man so wounded would ever be able to fight again, but the records do show that he was later discharged, in good health, from a base hospital.

And so it proved throughout the test series. Mortality dropped. Post-operative complications were substantially minimized where they were not eliminated altogether. Shock—and shock deaths—became a minor worry where once they had been a major surgical problem, aggravated by the intense cold in which the fighting was conducted. Long before the test was completed, the surgeons at the test hospital were fully convinced of the efficacy of the Vishnevsky method. Soon it was being adopted all along the Finnish front.

The Russians have not, of course, gone all overboard for this one particular type of anaesthetic procedure. They utilize many of the other types, general, spinal, and so on, where they think them preferable. But their early reports were so enthusiastic, that British surgeons greeted the entire matter with cautious skepticism. The great British bible of war medicine, *Surgery of Modern Warfare*, edited by Hamilton Bailey and issued in sections during 1940 and 1941, contains no word along the lines of the Russian experience in its first articles on anaesthesia. In fact, the writer of its special article on this subject permitted himself to say that "spinal and local anaesthesia is seldom indicated in operation for war wounds" and that "spinal analgesics in the ratio of ten per hundred are more than enough for the field hospital stock. Similarly, the stock of local analgesics should be comparatively small."

A year later, in completing the appendix to the fifth and last section of the massive volume, Dr. Bailey himself noted and praised the work of Vishnevsky, Novikov, and Pshenichnikov. Since then, the new methods have been receiving more attention from the British than was at first the case and more and more frequent reports of the use of the same or essentially similar local anaesthetics are being heard.

In the United States the new Russian method is comparatively unknown. This may, in part, be due to the fact that there is less interchange of surgical and medical knowledge between this country and Russia than has been the case with England. In larger measure, however, it may be because of the fact that, under domestic conditions and under foreign war conditions in the months immediately following Pearl Harbor,

American methods have proved more than ample for the task. American surgeons have shown the same tendency away from a complete reliance on general anaesthesia for most major operations, but this trend, in our country, has taken another direction.

The Navy, for instance, uses local anaesthetics, but not the Russian methods, for a great many operations on almost every region of the body. It has, however, tended to prefer spinal anaesthesia, using it in a two-to-one ratio as compared with local drugs. Spinal anaesthesia uses the same drug the Russians used, but in far more concentrated doses. As the name implies, the drug is injected into the spaces between the vertebrae in the lower part of the spine. Thus the entire lower portion of the body, from the diaphragm down, may then be operated upon without pain. On shipboard, where fully trained medical assistants may not be available to the surgeon, where space is limited and where fire dangers prohibit the use of gas anaesthesia, spinal injections are considered ideal. However, they are not advisable in cases of shock, particularly where much blood has been lost.

The Navy's favorite in these cases is intravenous anaesthesia with the use of a new drug, potenthal sodium. While of great use under all conditions, this drug is particularly suitable for use on shipboard. It produces rapid anaesthesia with quick recovery. It may be administered by people with only limited training. It is fireproof and non-explosive and it requires nothing more than an ordinary hypodermic syringe by way of equipment.

When a man is brought into the sick bay, the surgeon inserts the needle of the syringe into a vein in the patient's arm. The man is told to count slowly and the fluid is pumped drop by drop, in time to this counting, into the veins. Usually, before the man has reached a count of twenty, he has passed out completely and the operation may begin. Thus the dose is readily adjusted to the individual tolerance of each patient, since injection is halted when the counting stops.

As the surgeon proceeds with his operation, the needle is left in the vein. At the slightest sign of returning consciousness, an extra drop is injected by an attendant. This is sufficient to re-induce complete coma for an additional period and the surgeon can proceed without hurrying his work.

One of the greatest advantages of the intravenous method is the fact that the dosage is so closely related to the patient's needs. He returns to consciousness almost as soon as he is removed from the operating table and can thus co-operate in any later procedures.

Potenthal sodium is receiving ever wider use among the British armed forces, particularly for emergency operations at front-line dressing stations and near-the-front hospitals where its ease of administration and lack of after-effects are particularly valuable factors. But even in large hospitals where the availability of heavy equipment makes the choice of anaesthetic a wide one, the new drug is often replacing older and more cumbersome methods.

The effect of the improvements in anaesthetic techniques is hard to describe in terms of mortality. Certain it is that very few deaths will occur on the operating tables of this war which can be ascribed directly to the use of anaesthetics. But the most important factor of change has been that of lessened post-operative difficulty. No matter what the anaesthetic used, the wounded soldier can be certain that he stands a far lower chance of suffering, after the operation, from any of the numerous complications, from nausea to pneumonia, that once followed a large percentage of the operations performed under general anaesthesia in the last war.

Chapter XII

FLYING DOCTORS

"Never before have so many owed so much to so few."—Winston Churchill, acknowledging England's debt to the men of the Royal Air Force, September, 1940.

THE aviator is, without question, the heroic symbol of our age. He is the youth who does more than a man. He steps into a complex of machinery—wings, motors, guns, and instruments enough to make the mind swim —and he becomes part of that machine. More, the machine becomes part of him, an extension of his body that takes to the air, swings with incredible speed, sees over the horizon, sees even through clouds or at night, lays its destructive eggs just where he plans and then whisks him away from the scene with a zoom and a roar that terrifies all groundlings.

Try as we will to get used to the plane, it continually surprises and astonishes us by doing the impossible. Try as we will to look at the pilot as just a youngster, barely past his first shave, we find ourselves reverting to hero worship for these men who know none of the ties that bind the rest of us to earth.

Yet the aviator is a creature of whom it used to be said, "Nature never intended that he should fly." If he is a better man than we are, he owes the advantage only in the slightest degree to nature. For the most part he owes it to the doctors' defiance of nature—a defiance which first selects him from among the rest of us and then protects him, much to his annoyance, during every moment of his life.

It has been the doctor, the flight surgeon, who has taught man how to keep pace with his incredibe machine. Without aviation medicine, modern military flying would be virtually impossible. The cost of flying, even excluding combat losses, would be more than any nation could bear. Too many pilots and too many planes would crack up for the training programs and the plane factories to keep up with them.

In fact, that was exactly what was happening when flight surgery was first called into being, in 1915. In the early days, anyone who had the courage to fly did so. And it took courage, real courage, to get into the crates of bamboo and bailing wire that passed for airplanes back in 1912. It was only after the first year of the first World War that the various fighting nations began to examine their records of airplane failures. To the British in particular this examination provided a terrific shock.

The English airmen had been losing pilots almost as

fast as they trained them. Yet their planes were no worse—though no better—than those of their German opponents. That they knew, because they weren't losing their planes in combat. On the contrary, for every hundred pilots killed, that first year, only two were killed by Germans. Eight others died from defective equipment—when something snapped in the plane or when a motor coughed once too often. But the rest, ninety out of every hundred, died because of their own defects. Either they should never have gotten off the ground at all, or else they were too worn and tired or too nervous and emotionally upset on the day of their last flight.

The answer was obvious, after a year of needless casualties had pointed it out. Methods must be devised and tests set up which would eliminate the unfit-to-fly at or near the very start. And pilots must be cared for and watched regularly to make sure that they continued to be fit for flying duty.

Even so, the doctors didn't have an easy time horning themselves into a "purely military matter." One of the most spectacular leaders of aviation of that day thundered his formula, "I know perfectly well how to tell whether a man is a good pilot or not—if he goes up and breaks his neck, he's not a good pilot."

Luckily for the aviators, the doctors beat the "practical men" in the very first fight. They got their chance in 1916 and they made the most of it. Before another year had passed, they had beaten down the rate of pilot failures to a point where none could question the validity of their methods.

None, that is, except the doctors themselves. For from that day to this, the aviation medicos have been a most cantankerous sect, so in love with their own specialty that their idea of a really fine week has proved, time and again, to be a meeting in which each could denounce the methods of the others with the most profound scientific arguments. Put two flight surgeons together and you got an argument. Put three in the ring and you got three new theories.

Though the records of their meetings read like a long series of Donnybrook fairs, each marked many profound advances over the earlier tests by which they eliminated the unfit-to-fly. Their first tests were rule-of-thumb affairs. Some of them were way off the track, but others showed an amazing ingenuity which brought about results.

One of their biggest boners was the whirling piano stool. They used to put a candidate for flight training on a stool, whirl him around and then, if he became nauseated and vomited, they rejected him. Doctors now know that some of the best flyers in our air forces could never pass this test, for such nausea is a normal reaction.

Today, though, almost every test used to determine physical fitness for flying has stood up in practice and

flight surgeons are more worried about other questions
—particularly about anticipating the psychological reactions of their candidates for flight training. Their
physical tests, none the less, are so complex and so
thorough that they must still bear a fascination for the
rest of us who know only the ministrations of insurance
examiners.

Let's follow Joe Brown, one of several hundred
youths fresh from two years of college, as he turns up
all primed for flying at a primary training center. Joe's
first disconcerting shock is the discovery that he won't
get any attention from the doctors on his first day in
camp. They deliberately give him a twenty-four hour
rest, so that train fatigue shall not influence their examination results.

The next morning Joe starts through the meat-
grinder. First he gets a general physical survey; his
lifetime medical history is taken. Every infection, illness, and operation he has ever had (and will confess
to) is listed. Here the first filtering process occurs. Out
go not only all men over 200 pounds and all above six-
foot-two and below five-foot-four, but also every man
who fails to come within sixteen pounds of normal
weight for his height.

But Joe passes. He is neither too short to fit a plane's
controls nor so tall that he will get in his own way in
a narrow cockpit. Nor will they have to dump gas to
make way for Joe's weight. Joe goes on, to the eye

tests. Here he gets his first real pummeling. He's tested for near-sightedness, far-sightedness, and astigmatism. They then try him out for visual acuity, the ability to appreciate form, a mighty handy ability if you want to know whether that's a Heinkel or one of your own escorts on your tail.

Joe is seated exactly twenty feet from a test chart, the room is darkened, the chart illuminated, and Joe begins to read. If he can't read down to the second line from the bottom, out he will go. But Joe is normal. In fact, he sails right through the chart, right down to the smallest letters on the bottom line. They rate him 20/15, meaning that he can read, at a twenty-foot distance the line scaled for fifteen-foot reading. Joe begins to feel cocky.

But not for long. Next thing he knows they've got him up before a depth perception box. He's seated just twenty feet from a lighted box, with a window on its side. Through the window he can see two upright, black rods. The lights are so arranged that the rods cast no shadows which might otherwise guide him. One rod is fixed, the other movable by a pair of strings which are placed in his hands. Joe is told to line up the rods by moving the cords. And every time he does it, the doctor puts the rods out of line and makes him do it over again. The boy ahead of Joe fails to get within one inch of perfect alignment on the average of five trials. Home he goes.

But again, Joe does well. Some day soon his depth perception is going to prove pretty handy when he has to take a big plane into a landing on a small field.

Then they go to work on Joe's eye muscles, with a series of testing instruments. After about an hour of "fussing around," as it seems to Joe, they find that his muscles are in balance, neither too active nor under-active. Once Joe gets into a plane, where his bodily movements are restricted and where he will have to fix his eyes on fast-moving objects at quickly varying distances, Joe is going to appreciate that good set of muscles.

Right now, however, he's too busy. They've got him reading a series of colored charts, the pseudo-isochro-matic plates invented by a Jap named Ishihara. Each plate consists of a maze of colored dots. Some form just a crazy pattern. But others have the dots so arranged that a lot of one color line up in the shape of a numeral or letter against the rest, of another color, which form a background. If Joe were color blind, he wouldn't see the difference between the two shades of dots and he'd say that the plate had no figure on it. But Joe reads all the figures off, just like that. He'll be able to recognize the field boundary lights, navigating lights, and rocket signals and colored flags used for daytime signaling. And when he has to make his first forced landing, he'll know—from the color of the ter-rain—just what conditions he's going to meet.

Curiously enough, the air forces are beginning to loosen up their rules against color blindness a bit. Not for pilots, but for some types of observers. For a few years ago one observant flight surgeon had a strange experience. He took an officer friend of his up for a joy-ride. And the officer spotted camouflaged gun emplacements that the surgeon couldn't see. When they went to work on the man's eyes they found him badly color blind, so much so that he wasn't fooled by camouflage meant for normal eyes. Now, a few color-blind men are kept around by the air force for camouflage spotting, although most of this work is better done—when time permits—by using color-filtering cameras.

Finally, they test Joe for night vision. They make him stare at a bright light for three minutes. Then they put all the lights out except a dim one which the flight surgeon holds in his hand. If blinded Joe can see that light in three minutes, he'll do. If he can't, they may reject him. Or they may give him a high vitamin-A diet for the next few weeks and another chance. For lack of vitamin-A has been proved to be one cause of night blindness. This test is a rough one, good enough for the general run of flyers but nothing like the test Joe will have to pass, later, if he is to specialize in night fighting.

By this time the morning has passed and they lead Joe and the rest of the boys off to lunch. Joe notices that the group has shrunk perceptibly. He wonders whether he'll still be around by supper time.

On his return, they start on his ears. They play a record that doesn't make any sound. But wait—it does. It whispers. And Joe hears it at twenty feet. Hears it and repeats it to the examiner's satisfaction.

Then they try Joe for balance. First he stands erect, without shoes, with toes and heels touching. Then he flexes his knee backward to a right angle. Then closes his eyes thinking, "this is a cinch." The next thing Joe knows, he's flat on his face with an increased respect for the examiner.

On the next two trials on the right foot, Joe weaves just a little. Then on the left foot, he gets the hang of things—gets just enough confidence back to flop again on his last test. But he passes because he did maintain his position for fifteen seconds in better than one out of three trials on each foot.

Another test that gives Joe added respect for these strange doctors and their stranger gadgets is named after its inventor, Bárány. The Bárány chair is a sort of piano stool with a head rest holding the head forward at a thirty-degree angle, a foot rest, and a stop pedal. Joe gets in and is asked to fix his eyes on a distant point. Then they turn Joe around to the right, eyes closed, ten times in twenty seconds. The instant the chair stops, Joe hears the click of the examiner's stop watch and, obeying previous instructions, he stares straight ahead at the point selected before. A horizontal oscillation of his eyeballs occurs and it is clocked. Joe's lasted exactly twenty-five seconds, a second less than normal. But anything from 10 to 34 seconds would qualify, provided that it didn't vary by more than five seconds from the record made when Joe revolved in the opposite direction.

The test seems interesting enough, though rather pointless to Joe, until they tell him that it measures his ability to recover balance after a change of direction in the air. They also tell him that he'd better learn right now to trust his instruments more than his senses and they prove it by putting him back in the Bárány chair. Joe sits with his head on the rest and closes his eyes. They spin him to the right fast, then bring the chair to a dead stop. "Which way are you going, Joe?" asks the examiner. "Left," Joe answers. Then he opens his eyes to find that he has been stock-still since the first spin ended. Unless Joe is entirely too cocky to make a good flyer, he gets the idea at this point.

And so the day progresses. They go after the noses, throats, and lungs of the candidates. They throw out all sinus sufferers; they temporarily disqualify all diseased tonsil cases. Adenoids large enough to cause mouth breathing are taboo.

They take electro-cardiograms of the boys' heart actions. They take their pulses. They make the boys jump a hundred times on one foot and take their blood pressures before and after, and minutes after jumping.

And when they're all done, they have rejected any-where from a quarter to three-quarters of the group being examined. For every Joe who passes, some other boy is heart-broken to find himself "physically inade-quate"—often a boy who rated high in high-school and college athletics.

Yet the examiners haven't tried to keep the boys out. They've tried to pass as many as could be passed without wasting training on ultimate failures. For time has taught them that the worst thing they can do, for both the air-minded would-be flyer and for the air corps as well, is to train a man who hasn't got what it takes. Sooner or later he must be busted out—and it's better to break his heart than to have him kill one or a dozen trained men and wreck a few good planes, busting out the hard way.

The great failure of flight surgery—and a failure which the flight surgeons are the first to admit—lies in the inability, up to now, to apply equally exact and precise tests to the determination of psychological fac-tors making for success or failure as a flyer.

The doctors have done much in the way of learning how to detect personality traits leading toward success or toward failure. But their measurements are still a bit short of the ideal of accuracy and some failures that were not detected always crop up during primary training—and sometimes even at later stages.

How effective—and how ineffective—these tests (or
estimations) are as a means of eliminating those with
pre-conditions for psychosis or neurosis is shown in
some statistics cited by Lieutenant Commander R.
Barry Bigelow of the Navy's Pensacola Training Station. Dr. Bigelow reported that during the first six
months of 1940, with between twelve hundred and
nineteen hundred average membership in the student
corps, only twenty-four pilot candidates were referred
for neuro-psychiatric consultation, including all the
more obvious psychiatric disorders developed during
training.

That doesn't sound bad to you or to me. But it
sounds terrible to a lot of flight surgeons and they have
been busy as bees trying to do something about it. For
instance, the following case is the sort of thing that
makes men like Bigelow mad with themselves for a
week. A student reported to Bigelow on his own initia-
tive and made the following statement:

"I have been living in a daze all my life but I
scarcely knew it myself until the last few weeks. I
don't seem to know any more what is going on at the
time or in the present but then it seems that I can only
know things as though they were in the past. And
then it seems that I could tell what was going on in the
future, too.

"It seems as though I was day-dreaming and night-
dreaming at the same time. Just about everything that

happens to me, I am in a daze and then I recall what was supposed to happen and it leaves my mind blank.

"In my dreams people are talking about me all the time. They give the thoughts as well as the actions. It goes on except when I can realize what goes on around me, and if I keep talking fast, it is not so bad, but it makes me all mixed up. I don't feel like flying because I'm too mixed up. Anything that requires concentration seems to make it worse. My trouble is this living in the past and in the future at the same time."

A gross case of schizophrenia, you may say, which obviously should have been spotted long ago. Yet only a few weeks before this candidate had passed the most rigid of exams. For his condition was latent, though the pre-conditions for his breakdown probably were with him for many years. It took the severe strains of aviation training to bring them to their full foul blossom as obvious insanity.

Somewhat more frequent are the men with paranoid trends, though here again we must never forget that the number who get past the first medical sifting are few indeed. And those who do get by show themselves quickly, as they run into difficulties in training. Their paranoid tendencies manifest themselves most often as projections of these difficulties. Some believe that their flying is excellent, but that they are the object of the personal prejudice of their instructors who —the paranoids think—are unwilling to admit their own inferiority. Others convince themselves that their flying is poor because they are being refused a fair opportunity to improve it.

Whenever these distortions of reality are well marked, the practice has been to discharge these men from the air service as incapable of successful adjustment in this field.

For instance, there was the student who was sent to Bigelow because he had failed two final check-tests in primary planes. "His record," the surgeon states, "up to this time has been good, unusually good, and he was regarded as good officer material. He stated that he had always succeeded with ease in anything he had undertaken but became bored, lost interest and quit when his work presented no difficulties to him. He wondered whether this tendency was not manifesting itself in his flight training.

"He described various difficulties with his girl friends, to one of whom he had been devoted for years. He had broken off the relationship with her because he thought she was too stubborn to be compatible with him. He described many instances of over-reaction to real or fancied slights or injustices.

"He continued to have difficulties with his flying and a few days after the interview informed several instructors that they were too timid and too conservative and were criticizing his flying because *he* did not suffer from these disabilities."

In civil life, cases such as these might be dealt with by psychiatrists as individual problems. Often patient work may eliminate the attitudes which lead the paranoid to see his own failings in terms of the antagonisms of others. But in military aviation, the flight surgeon must consider the nature of the life each student will be expected to lead. He cannot trust any man's life—nor the country's safety—to the sort of individual who will break down under stress. Particularly in aviation so much depends upon the individual staying power of each man's nervous system, that only the best systems can be allowed to continue in the service.

In many another case, however, the psychiatric officer's duty is not so much to eliminate men as to explain and adjust difficulties. Yet always his criterion must be not the personal welfare of the individual under examination but rather the welfare of those the man will work with after he gets past his training and into active service.

A number of men in Bigelow's groups at Pensacola developed so-called anxiety states. These appeared to be related closely to fear of flying and were characterized by attacks which did not occur while the subject was able to secure leave of absence or was otherwise prevented from flying, indicating clearly the nature of their source and cause. Typical is the case of a student interviewed because, having completed above twelve hours of dual instruction, he was not regarded as safe for solo flying. He made the following statement:

"During the last couple of weeks, I have had some indigestion. I sit down to dinner and take a couple of bites and then I get dizzy and short of breath and it seems as if my heart begins to race at the same time. I have had the same thing happen to me when I was trying to drink a beer, too. Lately, I have begun to wake up at night and right away I would begin to try to fly that airplane in my own mind. Then, when I am flying, it seems that the ground hypnotizes me so that I can't tell what I am doing and one day I will level off high and the next time I will fly right into the ground and it just seems that I can't figure out what I am trying to do."

This particular man was relieved from duty and from the service. But in other cases, not so marked, the psychiatrists have been able to guide the student past his initial difficulties. In one sense, the primary training period serves as a testing ground for the nerve systems of the men. Men who cannot take the strains of modern flying in their stride usually show their weakness soon enough to be eliminated during primary training.

This is one reason—though only one—why no softening up of such primary training is considered. The course, both in Army and Navy centers, is intensive and difficult. It involves many subjects which are completely new to most students. It demands their most strenuous efforts over six or seven months followed by further training of indefinite duration under service conditions.

The great majority of the students are earnestly determined to succeed. When difficulties arise which threaten to lead to discontinuance of their training, it is but natural that they should respond to these with tension and anxiety.

It is not that they do respond, it is rather the way in which they respond that counts. For the ones with constitutional weaknesses—the ones who will break down sooner or later—respond now with pronounced reactions, clearly evidencing their heretofore unseen unfitness. For them, the primary training proves to be another test—and one which they fail.

But the more stable men respond with more moderate evidences of anxiety. Most of them find their own ways of licking their problems. Many help each other out. And others profit greatly from discussion with the psychiatrists. Once they lick their nervous troubles— their natural nervous troubles, under the circumstances—they are better fortified to withstand the still greater strains of actual combat flying. For now they need no longer fear their fears. They have licked them once; they know what they are like and they can lick them again, on their own.

One of the minor anxiety states which even the best

students sometimes fall into is known, colloquially as "checkitis"—a fear of check flights and check pilots. Here the men must be convinced that they can think of whatever they decide they want to think about. Instead of letting their fears make them concentrate on the check pilot sitting behind them, they begin to feel that they can concentrate, at will, on their flying rather than on the man who checks them. And beginning to feel that way, they acquire the ability. Often a single friendly talk from an older man will snap a good student out of a streak of "checkitis" and back into the normal progress of his flight training.

When the psychiatrists find their charges working out their own solutions of their problems (rather than explanations of their failures), they encourage them no matter how bizarre the solution itself may seem. One man was called to the attention of his flight surgeon because he was making seemingly strange motions on his walks to and from classes. But when he explained that he was practicing banks and turns at every turn of the paths, his adviser not only commended his actions but began to teach the same trick to others. For such practice is the surest way of converting the merely learned responses of flying into conditioned reflexes which free the flyer's mind for attention to other matters, equally important.

Thus do the flight surgeons perform the most basic, prosaic, and yet, most important part of their work—

the preventive medicine that selects, from among hundreds of thousands of eager young Americans, those who are best fitted by nature to meet and conquer the challenge of their own machines and of the best the enemy can offer.

Yet, after all the selections have been made, after all the pilots and observers and bombardiers and navigators have been trained, the flight surgeon is still around and still busy. For there is a second and most vital phase of his work, without which no air force could survive. Under the clumsy name of "care of the pilot" the flight surgeon finds himself performing the combined services of doctor, dietician, father-confessor, brood hen, and outlet-for-pent-up-emotions. Assigned to a squadron or flight of planes, he must exercise all the arts of diplomacy if he is to succeed in carrying on his work, in all these capacities, effectively.

Take our friend, Joe Brown, whom we met a few pages back getting his first taste of military life on the Bárány chair. Joe today is a newly graduated pilot, a young, healthy, intelligent individual who combines a high pride in his newly won wings with a profound respect for his new skills and for the machines he has learned to control.

Joe is healthy. He won't get more than his fair share of the ordinary illnesses and accidents which all soldiers are subject to. But his physician-in-waiting, his squadron flight surgeon, knows that Joe must be watched for more than colds and belly-aches. Joe is subject to a whole series of special, occupational difficulties. His occupation is a sedentary one—though it may seem strange to us who don't fly to think of a man who wings through the air at five miles a minute as being sedentary. But though Joe sits for long hours at his work, he is subject to strains of a nervous sort that he cannot be expected to withstand unless he is in tip-top physical and mental shape. It is up to "Doc," his flight surgeon, to keep Joe toeing the performance mark. Failing that, it's up to Doc to ground Joe.

Now when you set up a relationship of this sort you're heading right for trouble, unless your doctor is a master of human relationships. Joe and his fellow pilots are young men, intensely in love with their work. If they hadn't been, they would never have won their wings. Since Joe is a well-balanced individual, he has always looked upon his flight surgeon as one of the boys—a bit older than the rest of the men, but a good hand at poker and not at all bad at flying.

But then Joe runs into a stretch of active duty. Conditions require that he be sent aloft pretty often—and on pretty long flights. Joe finds he's not sleeping too well. It's too damn hot down on the ground, he tells himself. You wake up just as tired as when you flopped into bed. And the food has gotten worse. The rest of the men say it's all right, but Joe knows. Holy smoke, a man ought to know the food he eats. It's overcooked one day and undercooked the next. And the mail is being held up. Not a letter from home in four weeks. Sure, no one else has had any mail either. But you'd think a guy's girl would care enough about a guy to write him. She's probably checked him off, by now. A man can't even trust his own girl. That's a hell of a note. You can't trust anybody. Look at Cooky—here he had bunked with Cooky since the day they both turned up at Randolph Field. And only yesterday Cooky gets too damn smart and drops a decimal point somewhere in his navigation and they almost miss the station. If he'd trusted Cooky they'd be down at sea right now. There's no fun in flying if your own crew won't stick with you. But then who said there was fun in flying. Not when they keep you sitting at the controls night and day till your bones set and you can't stand up.

Joe is in a bad way. He's stale. Doc wouldn't be a flight surgeon if he couldn't spot Joe's staleness a mile off. Everything has piled up on him at once—overwork, overstrain, personal worries, loss of sleep, loss of appetite, loss of weight—and Joe is slipping into a tailspin that will crack him up fast unless he's grounded and grounded pronto.

But how's Joe going to feel when Doc tells him he's stale? How is he going to take the idea that he hasn't been quite as good as the next man? That isn't the case, but Joe will see it that way, unless he's handled just right. How is he going to feel towards the man who not only sets him down on the ground like an old cripple but cuts his flight allowances by doing so?

That's where Doc's tact and diplomacy are going to come in handy. Long before his charges become stale, the flight surgeon must have won their confidence and friendship. Even when they are mad at their best friends, even when they think their best girls have deserted them, they must still think Doc is an all-right guy. He can't treat Joe like a kid and get away with it. He must stand right up to Joe and let him have it head on. But if he has built up Joe's faith and trust in him in the months they've been together, Joe will take his grounding without more than a minor amount of kicking. And relaxation and change of pace will do the rest.

But playing nurse maid to a batch of flyers is merely the most time-consuming, not the most important part of aviation medicine. Military aviation must, inevitably, subject its flyers to physical stresses close to the limits of human endurance. In many respects the machine has outdistanced man and human factors are the limiting ones. Thus flight surgeons find it incumbent upon themselves literally to modify man, to raise human abilities in flight a peg or so and thus raise one nation's flying powers as compared with those of the enemy.

That's a tall order. But it has been met, time and time again.

One of the greatest advances in aviation was achieved when blind flying was perfected. Today the concept of blind flying is so familiar to all of us that we find it difficult to realize that the blind flyer is an aviator trained to ignore his normal instincts and reactions, a modified man who has been improved by aviation medicine in order that he may be able to do things that normal men could not normally do.

We owe the art of blind flying to the late Lieutenant Colonel David A. Myers, whose many years of patient research have revolutionized military—and civil—aviation.

Colonel Myers, then a young major, began studying the mechanisms by which man balances and orients himself, way back in 1926. The need for the ability to fly blind—that is to fly without reference to objects on the ground—had long been recognized. For aviation could not grow if every fog bank, cloud, and rain squall was going to wreck the flight.

But something interfered with every attempt to fly by instruments alone. It was Myers who first recognized what that something was and who first showed how to lick it.

First, he studied the senses by which man orients himself in his daily life. On the ground, subjected to strains and stresses which are normal for walking or the kinds of riding we do on the ground, Myers found our organs of orientation adequate. Between the sensations we receive through our ears, our balancing canals in the inner ear and our eyes—plus others from our muscles—we have little difficulty keeping oriented and in balance. We know whether we are standing or lying or leaning—we know whether we are moving and to a large degree how fast we are moving. We judge direction and distance with a fair degree of accuracy.

"But suppose," Myers reasoned, "suppose we take away one of our senses. What will happen then?" To test this idea, he blindfolded his friends and co-workers. The blindfolded men were told to walk in a straight line. But invariably they began to curve, either to the right or to the left. Once the curved path started they continued spiraling in a smaller and smaller radius. The more they turned the more they tended to turn, until finally they lost balance entirely and fell to the floor.

Now this is almost exactly what happens when a pilot gets lost in a cloud. Try as he will to fly straight, he will tend to wander to the right or to the left. Soon, still thinking he is flying a perfectly straight path, he will find himself in a steep spiral. His plane will finally go into a spin and out of control.

Then Myers turned to see what happened to birds when they were deprived of the sight factor in flight.

But, to everyone's surprise, even homing pigeons were found incapable of blind flight. When they encountered fog or clouds or when they were blindfolded and released from a plane, they simply set their wings for a glide and landed as fast as possible.

This maneuver makes good sense for birds. But it makes no sense at all for a flyer. His problem is to land only when he is ready to land and when the landing place is ready to receive him. When flying blind, without visual reference to the earth, the pilot must fall back upon his remaining balancing senses. But these have a nasty habit of lying to him.

We've come across one of these sense-lies before, when the Bárány chair was stopped and Joe Brown was fooled into thinking he was moving when he was really standing still. Nothing happened to Joe though, because the chair was firmly fixed to the floor.

But put Joe into a plane. Let him make a sharp turn. Being a good pilot, he will straighten out and level off. But the Bárány effect will occur and Joe will think he has turned, now, in the opposite direction. And this time he will compensate for the turn he didn't make. He will try to level off again. Actually he will turn out of level and wing again in the direction of his first turn. Pretty soon, the multiplication of Joe's reactions to these balancing illusions will have him flying way off course, flying sideways, and finally, going into a spin.

Now, with this phenomenon clearly established, Myers teamed up with another flyer, Major Ocker. Ocker was an old-time pilot and Myers tested him to see whether he could tell whether he was turning or sitting still. As long as sight guided him, he did all right, but blindfolded, he was just as bad as any novice.

Then Ocker had an idea. He built a view box, through which he could be allowed to see only a bank-and-turn indicator, the instrument that tells whether the plane is level or turning. He fixed the box so that he could light it or black it out at will.

With the light out, Ocker weaved and wandered in his test cockpit. He would make a maneuver and then overcompensate for it and presently he would be rolling the testing apparatus, in which he was seated, all over the place.

But then, he would turn on the light inside the view box. He would steel himself to ignore his sensations— those false sensations that had led him so terrifically wrong. He would concentrate on the bank-and-turn indicator and do only those things that were necessary to keep him flying on an even keel. Not the things he thought were necessary—for he knew now that he couldn't trust his senses when blind. Instead he did the things the instrument called for, no matter how these defied his sensations.

Myers, watching from the outside, could hardly believe his eyes. His friend, who a moment before was weaving like a Bowery drunk, now flew his test cockpit like the veteran he was. He went through maneuver after maneuver, and each time he straightened out and regained level flight and proper direction without any trouble at all.

Then they tried it out in the air. They put Ocker into a covered cockpit, with Myers behind him in a dual-control plane to grab the stick if the experiment didn't work. But Myers never had to touch the stick. Ocker had replaced his faulty senses with the foolproof senses of instruments. Blind flying had been achieved.

Soon it was improved by a whole series of new instruments. Radio guidance was developed so that a pilot could be kept on course by the sounds of radio waves beamed to fly along a given course. And the Link trainer was developed, the device which lets a student practice on the ground, under a closed, lightproof cockpit, until he learns the hardest lesson a man can learn, to defy his own senses and trust mechanical gadgets instead.

Once the doctors had started the thing, the engineers could carry it onward. They worked out whole systems of flying and landing and avoiding mountains, and telling how high you were above the ground instead of just above sea level. But the basis of blind flying had to be developed by the flight surgeon,

David Myers, before any progress could be made at all.

Blind flying, or instrument flying as it is better named, has brought in its wake new problems for the aviation doctors. Once man could fly by instruments, he could attack at night from hundreds of miles away, through clouds and storms if need be. But how to fight such attacks? Again the flight surgeons have had their part to play.

In this field the British have done most of the pioneer work. They have had to. Their work has followed the same two directional lines which characterize all aviation medicine, the lines of selection of those with the best natural endowments for the task at hand and the line of conditioning or modifying man to improve his performance over nature's best levels.

Let's watch Captain P. C. Livingston of the R.A.F. as he tests a group of pilots for night-fighting aptitudes. He leads six young pilots, fresh from their transatlantic training centers, into a darkened room. Each is seated on a chair whose special supports hold his eyes exactly one yard away from a central instrument. Each dons a pair of goggles—for the lights are still on—and each is given a board with a card clamped to it, and a pencil.

Then the lights are extinguished, the goggles are removed, and the students spend a final fifteen minutes adjusting their eyes to the pitch blackness. Meanwhile, in a low calm tone, the voice of Captain Livingston is heard.

"You are each seated," he tells them, "in front of a panel, which will be illuminated to reveal certain objects and letters, similar in character to the samples which have just been shown to you. There are four tests, each corresponding to a metal button on your boards and each test is exactly similar in technique. Each test exposes first objects and then letters. On the left space you will write the names of the objects you recognize. If you cannot do this, endeavor to copy what you see. On the right space, you will set down what you can detect of the letters. These letters may be set in abnormal positions. You may, for instance, find an 'E' with all the bars pointing upward instead of to the right. Copy it as you see it.

"Each test is of one minute duration. On each occasion the illumination will be slightly increased, till you reach the third test. Between this and the fourth test you will be subjected to one minute of glare from an electric lamp suspended above the apparatus. During this time you must not look at the lamp itself but directly below it."

As Livingston finishes talking, a faint glow becomes visible in the center of the room. As you peer, you make out the figures and symbols of the test. You realize then, as you struggle to see, what the young men with the busy pencils are up against.

All together there are thirty-two items to be identified. Thus a perfect score is recorded as 32/32. Only one man in about thirty will get between 30/32 and the perfect 32/32. About one man in forty won't get even two of the letters correctly. And the rest will range from very poor to pretty good.

When the British were first testing this device, they looked for a correlation between its results and the performance of their older night fighters. They found it, almost a hundred per cent. A man who was good as a night flyer, gunner, or observer, usually came out among the top third in a test. A man who had a poor record almost invariably scored less than 10/32.

That proved that they were on the right track, so they reversed the procedure. Flyers who couldn't pass the test weren't assigned to night work. And, as soon as the new men got into action in quantities their work provided the final confirmation for the Livingston tests. They flew better, bombed better, and fought better—for the very simple reason that they could see better in the dark.

After that, the device was used to test the effectiveness of medical plans for improving night vision. Was lack of oxygen, due to high flying, affecting night sight? They had but to test it, to find out. They took flyers who averaged a score of 23/32 at ground level and put them into a low pressure chamber where the air was as rarefied as it would be at fifteen thousand feet.

The same men, unchanged except for lack of oxygen, scored a rotten 6/32. From then on, night fighters were ordered to use oxygen as soon as they left the ground if they were going to fly over 9,000 feet.

They tried the same tests for dozens of other conditions. Some people said that vitamin-A would fix up anyone's eyes so that he could see in the dark. Maybe it would—and maybe it wouldn't. They fed vitamin-A diets to different groups. And they put a deep dent into a neat theory, if they didn't shatter it entirely. To vitamin-A's credit an improvement in night vision was recorded where the lack of "A" had brought about a falling off of this particular ocular ability. But some people who had plenty of vitamin-A still couldn't see worth a damn, once the sun fell. None the less, it was handy to know that "A" had a place in the aviator's diet.

They also tested men for dark adaptation. You remember that pilots must wear dark glasses for a while before taking the test. That is done so that their eyes can adapt themselves to the darkness. It is the same phenomenon you experience when you turn out the light to go to sleep. First the room seems pitch black. Then you distinguish a difference of tone near the windows. Then you pick out objects. If your night vision is good, you'll find after a while, that you can do quite a lot of seeing once your eyes have recovered from the bleaching effects of light.

But how long will it take to adapt your eyes to darkness? For one thing, it is going to take some people longer than others. That's another thing Livingston and other investigators have proved. But they don't select night gunners and observers by their speed of adaptation for a very simple reason. Any normal speed is too slow in an emergency. When Jerry comes over, you can't turn out the lights and ask him to wait till your eyes get used to the darkness. You've got to get up in the air all adapted to seeing him or you'll never stand a chance against him.

So once again the impudent doctors modify man, change him to meet new needs. They train night flyers to wear dark glasses. They used to make them sit in darkened rooms, but it is easier to wear dark glasses. And they give them luminous equipment, both in their planes and air stations, thus eliminating the glare of lighted instruments. In the air station a dark-spectacled fighter may play with phosphorescent cards or roll phosphorescent dice. Once in his cockpit, his adaptation to darkness will not be lost by looking at brightly lighted instruments. For night fighter planes have luminous dials that can be read in the dark.

By far the greatest achievement of aviation medicine has been the adaptation of flyers for high-altitude work. For, as the speed and climbing ability of planes has mounted month after month, the doctors were finding themselves hard-pressed by the engineers.

The engineers had by far the easier assignment. They simply had to teach an internal combustion engine how to breathe at high altitudes. The engine—like the flyer—needs oxygen and gets it from the air. As it moves into rarer atmospheres, it begins to starve for oxygen and soon it reaches its "ceiling"—a height above which it hasn't the power to pull a plane. Ceilings vary for different planes and different engines, but each has a limit beyond which it cannot go, unless you do something to aid it.

The something the engineers did was to introduce a supercharger. These complex devices are essentially simple in principle. They use a little of the power of the motor to scoop up large quantities of air and they compress that air. Then, when they feed it into the motor, it gets just as much oxygen from the air as it would get on the ground. It produces more power—far more power than the supercharger uses up. And its ceiling is upped five, ten, or fifteen thousand feet. In aerial combat those few thousand extra feet—or even a few hundred feet—spell the difference between victory and defeat. For the uppermost plane can dive at its opponent, gaining extra speed. The plane with the better supercharger usually wins in a dogfight.

That led some aviators to propose that the supercharger principle be applied to pilots as well. For the human engine—like the gasoline motor—can starve for oxygen. The aviators thought they could pump compressed air from tanks to the pilots and thus give them ground-pressure air at high altitudes. But the doctors scotched that one quickly. For air under pressure would simply "explode" the flyers' lungs. It would create ten times as much trouble as it would eliminate.

Instead, the doctors proposed to provide the flyer with better air rather than with more of it. Instead of feeding air containing 79 per cent nitrogen and 21 per cent of oxygen, they proposed to feed pure oxygen to the high flyer.

It was a beautiful idea, in theory. But it took many years to make it work in practice. They ran into all sorts of difficulties, before devices and techniques were perfected that would raise the flyer's ceiling up to where the plane ceiling had been raised.

Their first difficulty was the fact that the flyer doesn't usually know when he begins to need oxygen. For one thing, the rate of climb and the duration of exposure have quite as much to do with oxygen hunger as does the altitude. A plane that climbs faster will let a flyer get up higher before he passes out for lack of oxygen. And a man who might suffer no ill effects during the first half hour at twenty thousand feet may well suffer terrifically during his second half hour.

But even beyond these differences, there is the fact

that anoxia—the doctor's term for the sickness that follows oxygen starvation—is the sort of condition that masks its own symptoms. Above nine thousand feet, and increasingly so with the increase in height, the flyer finds his senses dulled. Above eighteen thousand feet, his nerve and muscle control begins to fail. Thus the ability to sense the situation he is getting into falls away exactly at the moment that the situation begins to become dangerous. And the ability to act to rectify the situation, by putting on the oxygen mask, is lost just when that ability would spell the difference between life and death.

To get around this problem, the air services of all nations now require the aviator to use oxygen equipment, even though it may be uncomfortable, long before the critical point is reached. Most pilots flying above twelve thousand feet are required and trained to use oxygen. And fighter pilots, whose planes climb as much as a mile a minute, often leave the ground with their masks on and the life-saving gas already flowing.

Another way of licking the oxygen problem is by the use of pressurized cabins. These have great advantages over the uncomfortable individual masks, since they permit of full freedom of movement and of work within the cabin. They simply maintain ground conditions—or conditions simulating any desired level—within the entire cabin. Since the pressure on the outside of the flyer (but within the cabin) is the same as that of the air he will breathe, you don't run into the difficulties that arise if you try to feed compressed air to a pilot whose body is seated in rarefied air.

Pressurized cabins are widely used for altitude flying, especially on big transport planes. But their military use is limited for one very sound reason. If the enemy gets his machine guns trained on a pressure cabin, he can rip it wide open in half an instant. You may imagine what would happen to the occupants then. They would not merely suffer from lack of oxygen, bad as that would be alone. They would rather experience a condition similar to the "bends" of a deep-sea diver who comes up to the surface too fast. For under rapid decompression the nitrogen in solution in the body (and particularly in the blood stream) goes out of solution and forms gas bubbles. They cause great pain and can bring on paralysis, convulsions, coma, and sudden death.

A similar condition occurs when men operate modern fighter planes which have high rates of climb. They climb so fast, in fact, that the flyer may be "decompressed" too rapidly in the same manner as the submarine diver is decompressed too quickly if he rises to the surface too soon and too fast.

During 1940 this condition was met with fairly frequently among English flyers and—with newer and faster-climbing planes coming along—the aviation surgeons were put to work to solve the problem. Once again they were asked to modify man to keep up with the improvements of the machine.

They found their solution rather more quickly than one might have expected. For they were able to fall back upon the work done by J. B. S. Haldane, ever since 1907. Haldane, son of one of Britain's greatest scientists and himself one of the great modern scientific minds, is particularly an authority on respiration. As such he has often been called upon by the Admiralty to investigate diving and submarine problems. Naturally he investigated the "bends."

Among the things that Haldane discovered was the fact that nitrogen bubbles would not be liberated unless the pressure was cut by at least one half. He therefore replaced the slow, steady ascent then prescribed for divers with a stage ascent, letting them come up for almost half the depth, then rest awhile, then halve the depth again, then rest—until they reach the surface none the worse for wear. It proved both faster and safer.

Haldane's formulas were not quite as simple as I have put it. They varied for other factors, such as the degree of nitrogen saturation. But suffice it to say that Haldane worked out tables that showed just how fast a man could be decompressed under any given set of conditions.

The flight surgeons who tackled the problems of

rapid climbing knew that they were concerned with nothing but a different aspect of the same problem Haldane had solved for divers. Haldane's solution, stage decompression, would work well enough for flyers, if time were not a great factor. For, if the flyer took his plane up a few thousand feet and then waited till he lost enough nitrogen he could go further up and repeat the performance. Eventually he would get very high without experiencing aero-embolism, the flyers' version of the "bends."

But you can't wait around in aerial combat. So the flight surgeons looked for some other way of turning the trick and eliminating nitrogen from the body speedily.

They found the solution to their difficulties in the oxygen apparatus they had developed to solve other high-flying problems. For oxygen inhalation has the effect of hastening the elimination of nitrogen from the body. In breathing air, the nitrogen in the air tends to balance the nitrogen in the blood vessels in the lungs. Thus elimination is slow. But when oxygen is breathed, the pressure of the nitrogen is all in one direction, out from the blood stream, through the lungs and away.

Very recently, therefore, the air doctors think they have solved the problem of aero-embolism without forcing the engineers to cut the rate of climb. All they do is make the flyer *start* using oxygen some minutes *before* he takes off on a flight. Thus, when he climbs fast, he does so in a nitrogen desaturated condition which permits him to get much higher up without feeling any ill effects.

How long the seesaw battle between the aero-engineers and the air doctors will continue cannot be predicted. Nor can we say who will finally win. But, up to now, it has been a toss-up. For every great engineering advance that produced a plane to tax the human body, the flight surgeons have been able to pull from their bag of tricks a bit of medical engineering that modified man, altering him in one way or another to meet the challenge of the machine.

Chapter XIII

BLITZ MEDICINE FOR BLITZ WARFARE

JOHNNY JONES is his name. He's twenty-three, has been in the Army eleven months, and is a corporal. He's bright and quick, with a touseled forelock that no military haircut can keep trained back and a smile that starts at the eyes and breaks all over his face if he likes you. He's healthy and he's happy and the only thing that gripes him is waiting around. His two desires are for letters from home and a chance to get on with the war and get it over with. You see, Johnny's got a girl back home, the sweetest, neatest, prettiest, smartest little girl in all Middletown. She's going to be proud indeed of Johnny when she hears about his being picked for officers' school. But, of course, she knew he would be.

That's Johnny Jones for you, one of the great American people's army. First he was one in a million. Then one in four million. Before he comes home, he may be one in nine or ten or twelve million. But to Mrs. Jones and to Janey Brown he'll always be that very special one in all the millions, their own Johnny Jones.

It didn't take Johnny long to discover, though, that he was many things besides Johnny Jones. In fact, in the last few months he's already been a dozen things, from number such and such on induction day, to a "dumb boot" to his first sergeant. To the Service of Supplies he's *another mouth to feed* and *two more feet to shoe.* He's a *trainee* and he's *manpower,* he's an *expeditionary force* and he's a *strategic reserve.* One of these days he's going to be a *landing force* and an *advanced element.* To the general's staff he's an *expendable.*

But to several hundred thousand assorted surgeons, doctors, orderlies, nurses, medical soldiers, and ambulance drivers he's another potential *casualty.* It is for Johnny Jones—for some unknown percentage of all the Johnny Joneses—that the greatest medical department in all history has spent millions upon millions for training, for hospitals, for ambulances and litters, for beds and instruments, for drugs and toxoids and serums. To protect and care for Johnny Jones, millions at home are going without their doctors. All the knowledge of all the ages, all the skills of a hundred years of medical leadership, have been mobilized for Johnny, the bright-eyed kid who is so many different things to so many people. There are surgeons waiting for whichever Johnnies may be hit, surgeons whom hardly any of the Johnnies could have afforded to hire in peacetime. For nothing is too good for Johnny Jones.

Yet between Johnny, just now hit, and all the miraculous techniques and devices and drugs of military medicine there stand a series of hurdles. These, too, are different things to different men. They are space: the space between the front line and the base hospital —space filled with men and munitions that must move unimpeded if the battle is to be pressed and won. They are enemy action: the long-range shells, the airplane strafing, the bombs and mines and booby traps that draw no distinctions between Johnny, well and with a gun in hand, and Johnny wounded and needing aid. They are also skill and training: the tough but tender hands of the litter-bearers who must navigate unarmed under fire to find the Johnnies and bring them back. Most of all, they are time. For Johnny's chance of survival depends as much on his making that journey from action to base in less than twelve hours as on any other single thing. In short, all the wonders of medicine will avail Johnny nothing unless a few everyday miracles of organization come to his aid. And that's where field surgery and the common, garden-variety medical private come into the picture.

Field surgery is a fusion of medicine and the military art. It is a compromise between the ideals of medicine and the hard necessities of battle, a compromise that varies with every army and every nation, with every war and even every battle. For there is a conflict between the purely military point of view regarding casualties and the purely medical or humanitarian viewpoint, a conflict which is resolved in different ways under different circumstances.

On the one hand, the commander of an army at war knows that his first duty is to fight to win. To do so, he must expend his men as well as his material. A good general will spend life cautiously, conservatively, never needlessly. But he will not hesitate to spend many lives when that is essential for his cause. To him, the first goal of the medical corps must be the achievement of recuperation for the largest number of wounded in the shortest possible time and the return of the injured to their regiments. From the "purely military" point of view it is actually more important to treat the lightly wounded than to save the gravely injured.

In sharp contrast stands the outlook of the medical man who, through a lifetime of civil practice, has been taught that the saving of life is his highest goal. It goes against every precept of his profession to neglect those whose lives might be saved simply in order to put others the more quickly back into the fight.

Seemingly, here is an irreconcilable conflict. Yet other factors enter the picture, particularly in a democratic army. For the wise general must consider the morale of his men and of the home front. Often these can be quite as important as any numerical factor of men available for fighting at a given moment. Experience has taught all armies that nothing so contributes to the collapse of combatant morale as a breakdown of the medical services, nothing so encourages a soldier to fight as the knowledge that he will get the best possible medical care if he is hit. Nor is anything more speedily effective in weakening the nation's will to fight than the knowledge that its men die as much of neglect as of enemy action.

The wise commander therefore modifies his "purely military" viewpoint and goes a long way toward meeting the "purely surgical" views of the medical men. He does so not on humanitarian grounds as much as on the sound grounds of military policy. He trades a little bit of quantity, in terms of men speedily restored to service, for a great deal of quality in terms of men and a nation willing to fight hard and well.

The exact point at which compromise is reached varies with the army and with the national ideal. The Japanese have managed to substitute a Shinto fanaticism for full medical services. The glory of dying for the Sun God Emperor replaces to some degree the will to live, among the severely wounded, though even the Jap generals dare not rely too much upon fanaticism. The Nazis have likewise tried to shift the balance of compromise toward the purely military side, although the attempt has stemmed largely from the racially fanatical Nazi party and has been opposed, to a degree, by the old-line generals who for once have joined rather than opposed the doctors. The fight came to the surface when the army proposed that racial theory be temporarily forgotten and that the remaining Jewish doctors be called upon to treat the wounded. To which the horrified Hitlerites answered that it is better to die untreated than to be defiled by non-Aryan medicine.

Some armies have shown a tendency to provide better treatment for the upper-class officers than for the plain privates drawn from the poorer strata. In the Czarist Russian Army and in the old Austrian Army this policy was justified on two grounds. "First," they said, "the poor devils are used to dying in peace and they therefore won't see anything out of the ordinary if we continue in wartime the distinctions of caste which we maintained before the fighting started. Secondly, it is obvious that a single officer is worth a score of cannon-fodder peasant soldiers; we must save the officer even at the expense of the soldiers as a plain matter of military economics." Just how well this policy —and all its associated policies—worked was demonstrated in the end by the disintegration of both armies.

In any army, such as our own, which bases its strength on the will of its people, such distinctions are manifestly out of place. The military leader may know that an officer or technician is more valuable than a common soldier. But he also knows that more valuable than either is the confidence of the army and the people in the effectiveness and the fairness of the medical arm. To retain this confidence no effort is spared, no expense denied as long as it will result in some strengthening of the effort to give the best possible medical attention to every man who may be wounded in action.

The Medical Corps of our Army has a long tradition of public service. Yet, in all our previous wars, it has suffered from the serious defect of lack of preparation, just as the Army as a whole has always before shown this same weakness. The medical arm of our fighting forces has had to be created anew every time we entered upon hostilities. By the time each war ended, our medical officers had learned their mission and evolved a form of organization well suited to the type of war that was being fought. But always, until now, this learning has been a process carried on *during* the war. Naturally, it was the wounded who bore the expense in terms of countless extra and needless deaths and endless days of pain and incapacitation. Once each war has ended, almost all of the medical men have returned to civil life. There they soon forgot most of what they learned in the field. They failed, invariably, to pass their knowledge on to the newer generation. With each succeeding war, the process was repeated.

But, with the first decade of the twentieth century, a change came about in our policy. An auxiliary medical corps was formed in the National Guard. We began to have part-time military doctors as well as part-time soldiers. And in 1908, years before any similar policy was adopted by any other branch of the Army, the Medical Reserve Corps was instituted. When we entered the first World War, in 1917, medical preparedness was further advanced than that of any other branch of the service. The policy paid handsome dividends in lives all through that conflict and enabled our army to avoid many of the costly errors that characterized the services of our allies.

With the peace, however, the old tendency toward disintegration of trained medical personnel again made itself manifest. From a peak, on Armistice Day, 1918, of over thirty thousand medical officers, the figures dropped rapidly, until by July, 1920, there were less than two thousand. But this time something else happened. The then Surgeon General, Merritte W. Ireland, established the Medical Field Service School and the Medical Department Equipment Laboratory at Carlisle Barracks, Pennsylvania. In this quiet, minor army post, set in the foothills of the Alleghenies, the tradition of medical preparedness was kept alive for twenty years.

The words "kept alive" are used advisedly, for often during those two decades it must have seemed to the rapidly changing commandants that they were entrusted with the care of a very weak child, and a stepchild withal. Half a dozen times the whole project was almost abandoned by merger with the regular Army Medical School in Washington. But somehow Carlisle

was each time given a new lease on its somewhat unhappy life and each year a few hundred more men of
the Medical Corps or the Medical Reserve took the
courses or attended the short-term summer camps. By
the time we entered the war, somewhat over twenty
thousand courses of instruction had been given. Over
sixty-six hundred reserve officers had learned at least
the rudiments of the hard-taught lessons of 1918. Today, of course, the Carlisle post is a flourishing institu-
tion, a field service "factory" that "processes" new
batches of army surgeons, veterinarians, medical soldiers, and other personnel every few weeks. Its grad-
uates are spreading the tradition in other army training
schools throughout the country. But much of the
strength of our medical services today will be owed to
those who hung on during all the lean years when an
assignment to Carlisle was not greatly to be distinguished from a polite form of exile.

The unromantic work of the Equipment Laboratory
is also paying dividends today. The work of the put-
terers who fussed, back in the twenties and early thirties, over new stretcher designs and low silhouette
ambulances, the work that seemed so pointless then,
today has given the Medical Corps a year's life-saving
lead. There may be some justification for the old saw
about generals always preparing to fight the last war
over again. But it becomes obvious to any visitor to

Carlisle Barracks that this does not apply to the Medical Department.

One of the most encouraging discoveries of such a visitor is to find, in the post bookshop, a whole shelf full of copies of *Field Surgery in Total War*, a book written by the New Zealander Douglas Jolly, after his service with the Spanish Republican Army Medical Corps. Even more encouraging is it to discover that this volume is a best-seller at Carlisle, a sort of Field Service bible. For nothing better evidences the breaking away of our medical services from the obsolete shibboleths of the last war and the adoption of new policies, fitted for the kind of field action with which a medical service must today cope. If the Spanish War taught us nothing else, it prepared a wide-awake Medical Corps for the changed conditions of modern warfare.

In the first World War, for most of the four years of fighting, the opposing armies were locked in the bloodiest of battles along fairly stable lines that extended from Switzerland to the English Channel. Wounds were almost invariably incurred at or near the front lines in an attempt to shift these positions a few yards in one direction or the other. For a fixed distance behind the lines, accurately measured for you by the guns of the enemy, you could not hope to carry on any extensive surgical work. Yet beyond the range of artillery fire, you could work with almost total certainty of freedom from enemy interference.

Thus, in World War I, on the western front where the French and British and American doctors learned their tactics, the Medical Corps operated in three distinct zones. The forward area or collecting zone extended from the front line for from four to seven miles. Here, within range of enemy fire, the main problem was the evacuation of the wounded. Litter-bearers took those too sick to walk back to the relay ambulance posts. From there they were rushed to the main dressing station or collecting station. The walking wounded too headed for these points and here both groups received their first *medical* attention, beyond the first aid administered them by the litter-bearers or company aid men. At the collecting station, only the most limited treatment could be given; it was principally a matter of providing such dressings and medicaments as would help the wounded to stand the evacuation journey.

Motor ambulances would then take the men beyond fire range to the casualty clearing station where the first real surgical interference would occur. Here the station surgeons would perform those operations which were most urgent. Often enough only a part of the surgical treatment would be given a man at the clearing station, that part which could not wait upon further evacuation without endangering his life or condemning him to months instead of weeks of convalescence. Here, for instance, wounds were cleaned and débrided, packed and bandaged, so that, after further evacuation to a general or base hospital, final and definitive surgical treatment might be given the man. Usually clearing stations were located on main lines of communication, so that speedy evacuation, preferably by train, could be used to take the men rearward.

Finally, in the rear zones, which in France covered the rest of the country, the ultimate surgical and medical treatment was given the seriously wounded.

In Spain, which proved to be the testing ground for all military theories, those who had come to think that this form of organization, so suited to the French front of 1918, would always be utilized were due for a series of rude shocks. The front proved to be far more mobile than twenty years previously in France. Often there was no real front at all, the armies mixing over a vast area of combat with only the most loosely defined lines. Aerial bombing quickly changed all zones into action zones. The matter of getting clearing stations out of range of shellfire became less and less important, for they would always be within range of airplanes. And the German and Italian airmen who flew Franco's planes soon demonstrated a positive affinity for the Red Cross. After the first few months in Spain no hospitals were marked as such for the simple reason that a Red Cross on tent or roof served as a plain invitation to bombing. Transport difficulties, in view of the limited road systems existing in Spain, further complicated operations. A station arbitrarily located by World War I standards might turn out to be inaccessible to the front once action began and the few roads filled up or it might find itself unable to evacuate its men toward the rear in anything like a reasonable period of time.

Thus, under the stress of a new kind of war, the entire problem was re-examined and a new system of field surgery worked out. As Jolly described the Three-Point-Forward System, the criterion of location of hospitals and clearing posts ceased to be the factor of distance from the lines. Instead distance was translated, in each special case, into its time components. The functions performed by the traditional clearing station were likewise broken down into their components. Nearest the front lines was the classification post, to which all wounded were brought. Here the wounded were sorted, according to the urgency of their surgical needs.

The most seriously wounded, men with severe hemorrhage, abdominal wounds, severe chest wounds, some head wounds and cases of grave shock, were sent to the Number I Hospital, so located that the time lag between wounding and hospitalization would never run to more than five hours. All other cases, except those of a trivial nature, were sent to the Number II

Hospital, located somewhat further toward the rear, with a time lag of not more than ten hours. The men who had slight but militarily incapacitating wounds were sent directly to evacuation hospitals, still farther back but not more than eighteen hours out of the zone of fighting. To these hospitals were also sent the evacuees of both the Number I and Number II Hospitals.

By thus breaking down the functions of the various hospitals the Spanish Army Medical Service obtained a number of advantages both in terms of better medical treatment and from the viewpoint of tactics. The most seriously wounded, who were brought to the Number I Hospitals, gained that most valuable of all elements, time. The advantage of this gain was not always apparent in terms of statistics and, for a time, the advocates of the Three-Point-Forward System were hard put to justify this phase of their work. For in some instances, the mortality rates at forward hospitals actually rose in direct ratio to the hospital's nearness to the scene of fighting. When, however, it was observed that a larger portion of the men who would never have survived a long journey—of say ten hours or more—did survive to enter a seven-hour-distant hospital, the reason for this apparent rise in the death rate became clear. Instead of falling back to older methods, the Spanish practice at this point was to move the Number I Hospitals still closer to the front. When this was done, a rise in the recovery rate occurred. In

Jolly's own experience, the recovery of severe abdominal wounds rose from thirty per cent to nearly sixty per cent when the time lag was cut to five hours from an original ten.

From the viewpoint of tactics, the Three-Point-Forward System serves greatly to increase the flexibility and mobility of the entire Field Medical Service. Under any system that puts all men, irrespective of wound severity or the character of their injuries, through the same clearing hospitals, a change in the time lag from the front necessitated the simultaneous movement of the whole hospital unit with a consequent disruption of service during the period of movement. This disruption was minimized, in Spain, by moving only one hospital in the chain at a time.

The change could be effected by either of two methods. One procedure was to detach, from the Number II Hospital, a complete surgical team and send it forward as a hospital group to form a new Number I. The old Number I Hospital then became Number II. The surgical teams from the old Number II came up to the new location one by one, as the number of cases in the old hospital decreased. As each Number II team arrived, the corresponding Number I team was released to move forward. Thus the shift was effected with virtually no loss of operating time and with no unnecessary shifting of the wounded. The matériel and the general personnel at the old Number II location would be held in reserve for another such move forward or, if the need rose, as often it did in Spain, for a reversal of the shift towards the rear.

Another method was to leapfrog the entire Number II unit over the Number I Hospital, reversing their numbers and function. While sometimes necessary, particularly in reverse action during a retreat, this proved to be the less desirable of the two methods, for it involved a greater disruption of service and it reversed the functions of the surgeons, so that Number I specialists had to do Number II work until a gradual shift could be effected.

The key to the entire Spanish system lay, obviously, in the maintenance of mobility. Such mobility was achieved by setting up basic mobile units, groups of men and equipment which always moved together. The basic unit was the self-sufficient Mobile Surgical Team, consisting of fourteen persons and always regarded as a fixed entity. It included a surgeon, an assistant surgeon, two anaesthetists, two operating theater nurses or orderlies, two general orderlies, three drivers who doubled as sterilizer operators, one electrician, and two ward nurses or orderlies. If the unit operated at an advanced classification post, its surgeons were men of general experience. Specialists in abdominal work usually were assigned to Number I Hospitals while specialists in chest, jaw, brain, and fracture surgery were allocated to the Number II Hospitals.

Each unit had two vehicles, a surgical lorry or "auto-chir" which carried all the surgical equipment, sterilizers, operating lights, operating tables, generator, etc., and an ambulance. This latter vehicle was used to move the majority of the personnel when the unit shifted location. When stationed at a hospital, the unit lent its ambulance to the nearest evacuation group, so that it would be utilized as much as possible but always be available for an emergency movement of the hospital group.

At a Number I Hospital, the number of Surgical Units varied from two to eight. These were supplemented by a *Triage* team consisting of two medical officers plus the necessary clerical and nursing staffs to organize the reception, sorting, and first-aid treatment of the incoming wounded. Pharmacists, blood-transfusion officers, and cooks and kitchen help were also added, each function being carried on by a unit which arrived at the hospital in its own vehicles with all its necessary matériel. The basic Surgical Team, however, was the all-essential. Without it, no hospital could be established. With it, treatment of the wounded could speedily begin, often within an hour of its arrival.

The real test of this system came when the Loyalist Armies were in rapid retreat, from March to October, 1938. The retreat was in two phases, interrupted by a counter-offensive which eventually failed. Thus every type of action, from advance to chaotic falling backward, was met by the surgical services. The small mobile units were able to hang on longer and then to retreat successfully under conditions that would have crippled large hospitals of the type used in France in 1917. During the counter-attacks, leapfrogging kept the hospitals within a close time-distance from the advancing front lines. At one point, a complete Corps Hospital Section and several surgical teams moved five hundred miles from quiet Badajoz Province to the field of violent action in the north. The journey was made in only three days and a few hours after their arrival they were dealing with major casualties.

Except for one short period, when the flooding of the Ebro River interrupted and delayed the movement of casualties, a time-lag of under five hours for the most urgent cases was well maintained, during both forward and rearward movements. In no small measure this was due to the courage and devotion to duty of the ambulance-corps personnel, yet neither courage nor devotion alone can account for the achievement. This was recognized by all armies when they began to study the records of the Spanish Civil War. While that first fight against the Axis served Hitler and Mussolini principally as a testing ground for new methods and new machines, it has brought an unexpected series of benefits to the United Nations, not the least of which is a radical departure from the Field Medical Service viewpoints of earlier days.

Neither the United States, Great Britain, nor Russia have adopted the Three-Point-Forward System in toto. To do so without regard to circumstances would, in fact, negate the all essential principle upon which the Spanish system was based. For the Three-Point System is an adaptation of medical field service work to one particular variation of the new kind of warfare. The flat terrain of the Russian steppes or the island fighting of the Solomons naturally demand variations of equipment and procedure to meet the vastly different conditions of these battlefields.

The United Nations of course are infinitely richer in medical manpower and in equipment than were the blockaded and matériel-starved Spanish Loyalists. The Russians have their ambulance tanks, equipped with trapdoor floors, that can run their protective bodies over an injured man and bring him safely through a hail of fire. They have their fleets of ambulance planes that, in certain circumstances, bring even the surgical hospitals of the large interior cities within a safe time-lag distance of the front, for the most serious cases. Our Marine Corps has its amphibian ambulances: armored, tank-like vehicles that can move with equal facility through a jungle path or over a wide ocean lagoon. Our Army has its fleets of evacuation ambulance planes, its scores of specialized, motorized laboratories, its mobile operating rooms, and its cross-country ambulances and hospital units.

Yet, for all our growing wealth of equipment, the men who guide our Field Medical Services can never forget that war is a matter of being ready for the unexpected. Supplies in wide profusion are great things to have, but the men who are taught to use them must also know how to get along when the transport breaks down, when isolated and surrounded, when the only drugs you can count on are the ones you and your men carried in with you. The Medical Corps is prepared, as must be any branch of any army, to live off the land and to utilize every makeshift when and if the need arises. Wherever possible, every last light and scalpel, every final splint and pill will be where it ought to be when the wounded first trickle back of the lines. But the men who run our medical services know that sometime, somewhere, more often than they would like, the supplies will not all get through.

To eliminate difficulties as they arise is the common triumph of peacetime engineering. But the victories of war, including the medical victories, come to those who know how to foresee shortcomings and how to get around them in advance. In respect to medical supplies, the army follows two related techniques: it first makes certain that a few, all-essential facilities come through for the wounded no matter what, and then it teaches everyone concerned with front-line work how to get by—and get by well—on makeshifts.

To list all the hundreds of such makeshifts would be an impossible task. For one thing, many of them are military secrets and others are known only to those specialized medical troops who will be called upon to use them. Sometimes, in fact, several devices have been invented, each a step further away from the standard Government Issue equipment, so that medical-aid troops can utilize whichever of them proves most handy to concoct under any conceivable circumstances. There is, for instance, the standard Army Service Litter. This consists of two poles of wood or aluminum, with attached folding rests which serve as short legs when the litter is put down. The poles slip through two tunnels sewn into a heavy canvas. Two cross bars fold out of the way when the litter is closed for storage or transport. A twist of the wrist opens the device and the folding cross bars effectively stretch the poles apart to form a canvas bed.

Wherever possible, a wheeled litter-carrier supports the stretcher, jinricksha fashion. This piece of equipment likewise folds for easy transport, opening to form an easy riding, easily drawn two-wheeled cart-chassis that provides a smooth, well-sprung carriage for the litter itself. When these are not available, or when they cannot be utilized because of the roughness of the terrain, other devices may come into play. The Cacolet adopts the standard Service Litter for horse transport. Two types are used, one carrying a single man, the other supporting two men on either side of the horse or mule. Failing this, the horse-drawn Travois may be used. Here two long poles are attached like shafts to either side of the horse, their free ends dragging along the ground. Cross bars hold the poles parallel and support the regular or improvised litter. Such a device serves to extend the ability of a fixed number of medical troops to evacuate the wounded, since only one man is required to maneuver both horse and patient.

Usually, however, four men will make up an evacuation team. Loading the wounded man onto the litter, by a procedure carefully routinized and endlessly drilled to minimize discomfort for the casualty, the litter team will break step and carry the man off, one soldier holding each pole-end. Even the act of breaking step is carefully calculated. It serves to minimize the jogging incident to fast litter travel over rough ground.

But suppose no litter is available. In that event the memorized first-aid manual tells the wounded man's companions how to improvise a litter in half a minute. One procedure calls for a blanket and two poles, the first coming from a soldier's pack, the second being cut from the first tree, if not otherwise available. A few pins are usually handy to help form a tube of the blanket, through which the poles may be slid. Failing these, the men may loop cartridge belts over the poles and lay the blanket over these improvised bed-springs. Lacking all these, another procedure is suggested. The overcoat of one of the men is taken off and turned inside out. It is buttoned and thus forms a tube. Rifles are slid through this tube and through each sleeve of the coat, forming a thoroughly practicable stretcher that will support the weight of the wounded man. Lacking even the coat, the medical-aid men know how to turn the same trick using two standard army shirts.

Seldom indeed will the last procedure—nor most of the other makeshifts—have to be called into use. But against the day when they may be needed, all men are trained to use them. More important, they are trained to think in terms of improvisation, so that they may go well beyond the suggestions of the manual to meet any situation that may arise.

Some things, however, cannot well be improvised. To make sure that these get to every fighting man, they are made a part of his regular battle equipment. In fact, the soldier who neglects to don his First Aid Kit is likely to be more severely disciplined than the one who fails to clean his rifle. Certainly both endanger their own lives and those of the men with whom they work to an equal degree. In the last war, the principal item in the kit each soldier carried was a bandage, by means of which he might limit the contamination of his or his buddy's wound, reduce bleeding, encourage clotting, and, in general, make it possible for the wounded to last until real first aid reached them. To-day, however, these kits contain two additional items of major importance. One comes in a small, tin slide-cover box and consists of twelve tablets of a sulfa drug. The first of these tablets the soldier takes as soon as he is wounded. Others are sufficient to serve, at three- or four-hour intervals, for nearly three days. The second new item is an envelope containing powdered sulfa-thiazole. This the wounded or their comrades pour onto and into the wound itself.

These two drugs, together, have already saved many an American life, for unlike the old-time bandage, which only limited further contamination, these serve to prevent contamination from becoming converted into infection. Here we have the other face of the time-lag coin. On the one hand, every effort has been made to minimize the interval between the incurring of the wound and its definitive treatment in a hospital. These efforts aim at the goal of holding the lag to a *maximum* average of eight to twelve hours, for after that lapse of time the germs that contaminate every wound tend to overpower the body's defenses and cause infection. Once the spread of infection occurs, the surgeon's abil-ity to intervene is sharply circumscribed. His hope of successful intervention is cut to half or less, depending on the location, extent and severity of the wound. Even when he is successful in treating an infected wound, the patient may spend five, ten, or twenty times as long in reaching recovery. But given the sulfa drugs applied immediately after wounding, orally and directly to the wound, we substantially lengthen the golden period. The sands in the glass of life, which once flowed away in a few short hours, are now doubled or trebled. Men who would once have died in the field or succumbed on the way to the hospital, now come through in better condition and with vastly improved chances for speedy convalescence.

The medical troops have other means at hand for holding back the clock, though most of these cannot be included in the individual soldier's kit. Aid men carry morphine in measured-dose, individual containers, so that pain can be eased quickly in the field. This is not merely a matter of relief to the suffering, though that is undoubtedly important enough. Morphine, properly administered, serves to delay the onset of shock and to minimize its severity. Once again, the golden sands are multiplied.

Yet these and other procedures, such as the administration of whole blood or blood plasma to shock victims, are only of value provided the process of evacuating the wounded is eventually completed. They can compensate for delays in evacuation. They can extend the patient's ability to endure evacuation. But they cannot serve, in any sense, as a substitute for definitive surgical treatment. Thus a great deal of the Medical

Corps' development work, in recent years, has concerned itself with keeping medical transport facilities on a par with the rapidly developing military transport facilities.

These developments vary from the simplest of serviceable makeshifts, such as the quarter-ton jeep converted into a litter-carrier, to specialized evacuation equipment designed for service with special army units. One of the most interesting of the latter is the amphibious ambulance which accompanies marine landing forces. This is a combination tank-boat, equipped with caterpillar treads and capable of rapid travel on both land and water. Originally developed for trial in the Florida Everglades, these units have already proved their worth in several tropical battlefields. They are capable of taking the wounded overland, through swampy lowlands, across the beach, and quite a distance to sea, bringing the men directly to a waiting hospital ship without transhipment at any point on the trip.

The Russian Armies, confronted by problems which have differed in both type and extent from any met by their allies, have worked out numerous specialized devices for aiding the evacuation of their wounded. Before launching their counter-offensive during the winter of 1941, the Soviet Medical Services made special preparations to facilitate evacuation of the wounded under the severest conditions of storm and cold. To prevent frostbite they provided heated ambulances, fur and padded-blanket bags, improvised padded dressings to protect affected organs from the cold and frequent warming and feeding stations along ambulance routes. They have made extensive use of chemical heating pads, which can be utilized under the most adverse conditions. These are fabric containers holding a quantity of prepared chemicals which react to the presence of water by developing and maintaining substantial heat for several hours. The water itself need not be hot; even snow may be introduced into the containers.

Often the wounded had to be carried through vast snowy wastes, sometimes in the midst of blizzards and snowstorms which made the roads all but impassable. Despite this, through the entire winter of fierce action, the Red Armies had not a single case of a wounded man in transit contracting frostbite. Many men, of course, were frostbitten during battle. These were immediately dispatched to field or rear hospitals for treatment.

The Russians, too, have made great use of airplane evacuation, for which purpose they have had specialized fleets of hospital aerial transports. They have even maintained contact with guerrilla elements scores of miles behind the German lines and there are many authenticated instances of successful aerial evacuations of guerrilla fighters who were one day wounded as far back as the Pripet Marshes and found themselves, the next morning, in a comfortable bed in one of Moscow's large hospitals. Almost all the wounded from such besieged cities as Odessa and Sevastopol were evacuated by plane.

Our own Army is prepared to go even further along these lines, having set up an evacuation service that will take the more severely wounded directly across the Atlantic for treatment in specialized hospitals within the continental United States.

Back of equipment, of course, stands the factor of medical personnel. Unless these are available, in sufficient number and with ample training, the finest equipment in the world would be of little avail. In this respect, however, the American armed forces are particularly fortunate. Many of the figures concerning our medical services come under the heading of restricted data, but enough is known to show that the American soldier is getting and will continue to get far more and far better medical attention than any troops have ever received before.

There were, at the time of our entry into the war, some 180,000 physicians licensed to practice in the United States. Of these, nearly twenty-five thousand were absorbed into the armed services during 1940, 1941, and the early months of 1942. Plans published in 1942 indicated that this number would rise, by the turn of the year, to something over forty thousand. The process will continue during 1943, the rate of growth depending, to a degree, on the progress of the war and the severity of the fighting. Eventually, with an Army, Navy and Marine Corps of some 9,000,000 or more men, the armed services would need, it has been forecast, nearly one-third of all the physicians in the country and two-thirds of all those under forty-five.

Many of these doctors were not called up as individuals but rather by Base Hospital Units, formed of doctors and nurses who had practiced together in large general hospitals. Some of the larger hospitals have sent as many as five such units into the Army, completely organized for active service and already having the training and esprit de corps so essential to successful military service. Many of these groups represent the continuance, in reserve, of units first formed in the last war. Among them are included many of the most skilled surgical specialists.

The majority of physicians, however, enter the Army or Navy as individuals and are assigned to units first developed within the armed forces. Unlike the doctors of the last war, a large proportion of these men have had some military medical training. Many thousands have been in the organized reserve. Additional thousands have had at least a year in the Army, prior to our entry in the war. These, in turn, serve to cushion the training of the newly inducted, who get more time to learn the difference between military work and civilian practice than it was possible to give our physicians in 1917.

The students in the medical schools have been deferred from the draft to permit them to complete their training. Most of those in fit health will enter the Army directly from their graduation ceremonies, adding something over six thousand men per year to the medical forces. These younger men are best-suited, by physique and by the special training their modified medical courses are giving them, for active field service.

In general, despite the high caliber of the men who composed our medical forces in the last war, it may safely be said that the new Medical Services have the best-trained doctors this country has ever produced. Those who have long served with the regulars, have had larger bodies of men to work with, since 1933, than any peacetime army of ours has ever had before. Their experience has been augmented by work with the Civilian Conservation Corps. The physicians drawn from civil life have, for the most part, come through the medical schools during the last twenty years, a period during which medical education itself has reached a new high plane. Our older men, including many of the specialists, have as a group won a pre-eminent place for American medicine since the last war. Undoubtedly they will be hard put to produce such giants as Cushing and Crile, but the average doc-

tor in the Army today is measurably better equipped
by training and experience than was his average predecessor in 1917.

At the time of writing, it is yet too early for statistics
to demonstrate conclusively the medical advantages
which our soldiers enjoy over their fathers in the last
war. The defensive actions in the Philippines, ending
as they did in siege and final surrender, have provided
only the most sketchy of figures. We do know that the
Medical Services worked—and worked well—to the
very last. We do know that many of the new techniques proved themselves in the field. But the nature
of the action and its unhappy outcome will probably
make statistical conclusions impossible, even after the
war is over.

In Hawaii, both the Army and Navy Medical Services scored phenomenally in terms of recovery rates.
Never has so large a body of wounded shown such
freedom from infection. Never have *such wounds* resulted in so few amputations, so few permanent inca-
pacitations as were achieved at Pearl Harbor. Never
have such severely wounded men been able to return
to duty after so short an average interval, nor have
they ever before returned in such good health. But
Hawaii was a special case, if ever there was one. After
a single attack, the medical forces were able to work
free of enemy fire. The climate was ideal. The scene
of the attack was such that large hospital facilities and

the medical forces of the entire Pacific Fleet were available for treatment, plus the local Army and civilian forces. Ninety-six out of every hundred wounded men who reached a hospital survived—only four died.

The British, on their home front, have likewise provided no figures that might be considered typical of the operation of medical forces in severe modern war. Their problems, though acute enough, to be sure, were nonetheless not of the sort to be encountered on the field of battle. The victims of the bombing of the British cities presented a special problem virtually unknown in the last war and one concerning civil physicians rather than the military forces. While their treatment taught us much that is hopeful in respect to many of our newer drugs and techniques, it was still no measure of field service conditions.

The British experience at Dunkirk comes closest to providing such a measure. Certainly much was learned about mobile hospital work, blood tanks, tetanus, and a host of other things, during the bloody retreat through France and Belgium. Yet this, too, was a special case. For some, at least, of the most severely wounded fell prisoner to the rapidly advancing Nazis and all of the rest were evacuated by boat for treatment at home. This evacuation, in some respects, militated against the men. Certainly the hazards of the rough journey across the Channel in small boats and without adequate preliminary treatment worked against many of the wounded. Whether the advantages of final treatment in British hospitals counterbalanced these shortcomings of the evacuation, cannot yet be determined.

In Libya and Egypt, once again, special factors make it difficult to see the entire picture. Much of the fighting was tank warfare. The British have evolved many new methods for the first-aid treatment of wounded tankmen and for their evacuation. Yet tank warfare in desert surroundings provides no over-all measure of the conditions large armies must meet before this war is over. The same is true of our battles in the Solomons and in New Guinea. The data is too incomplete and the conditions once again so specialized, that only a limited estimate of future results in large scale action can be obtained. In both cases, the limited reports indicate that the Medical Services are functioning well, that the wounded are being evacuated speedily despite the difficulties of terrain and the long distances over water to the base hospitals in Australia and elsewhere.

The latest reports from the Solomons, according to Admiral Ross T. McIntire, Surgeon General of the Navy, show a death rate among the wounded on Guadalcanal of less than one per cent, only one seventh as high as in the last war. Here, however, climate and the absence of infectious agents, may partially account for the favorable figure.

The one battlefield to which we can turn for a complete picture of modern military medicine in all its phases is Russia. This would not have been true were we dealing with a Russian Army at the level of development of that of the Czars. But Russian military medicine has advanced in facilities and mechanization on a par with the other arms of the Soviet military machine. Russian civilian medicine is regarded, by qualified physicians, as at least the equal of our own. In certain specialties, the Soviets lead the world. On the average, they certainly compare not unfavorably with our own Medical Services. The socialized nature of Russian medicine does, in fact, give the Soviet army one great advantage over both our own and that of the British, for Soviet doctors are already trained and organized in peacetime, to a far greater degree than our men, for the sort of co-operative work that army service demands. This is particularly true if comparison is made between the Russian doctor and our small-town, general practitioner. The self-reliance of our country doctors will undoubtedly serve them in good stead, but it does necessitate some adjustment of working habits and viewpoints to adapt these practitioners to the highly integrated methods of army work.

Despite these surface differences, the similarities between the Russian and the American Medical Services are so numerous that the results of their field surgery may be taken as measurably indicative of our own. Thus Soviet medical statistics provide a most hopeful index of what we may expect our own Medical Services to achieve.

During the first eight months of the Russian campaigns, more than one-half of all the wounded recovered sufficiently to justify their returning to action. This figure includes those wounded during the initial period when the rapidly advancing Germans were able, frequently, so to disrupt evacuation services as to increase greatly the time-lag factor. In the six-month period, from September, 1941, through February, 1942, including all the period of the winter campaign, the rate of recovery to fitness for active duty stood in the high sixties, two-thirds of all the men wounded in this period having returned to the front by the end of March, 1942. In the Finnish War, eighty-three per cent of all the wounded were restored to service before hostilities ended, an unprecedented figure in military history.

The Russians have had far fewer deaths from serious wounds than in the last war, their figures here reflecting directly the vast improvement in the medical arm. For overall, the nature of wounds in the current Russian fighting has been fully as severe as that of 1914-1917. The difficulty of treatment, in view of the vast areas covered, the winter fighting, and the changed conditions of evacuation induced by the airplane have further militated against the Russian wounded. Yet despite these factors, the Medical Services have so improved, in first aid, in evacuation technique, and in surgery and post-operative treatment, that substantial reductions in wound deaths have been achieved in almost every category. Thus, in a recent report, Deputy Commissar of Health Milovdov cited a drop in deaths from stomach wounds as compared with the first World War of more than thirty-three per cent. Head, jaw, and thorax wound deaths dropped fifty per cent. Spinal wounds, almost invariably fatal in the last war, showed a drop in the death rate of eighty per cent.

Over all, the Russian statistics show a death rate among treated wounded of only one and one-half per cent. While this surpasses anything ever achieved anywhere, except on Guadalcanal, it probably reflects the fact that, in the retreats of defensive warfare, not all the severely wounded are ever brought in to hospitals. Nonetheless, this figure speaks worlds for the caliber of the Red Army Medical Corps.

To all our millions of Johnny Joneses and to all those who wait for their return, these figures should indeed be encouraging in the extreme. Modify them as you will, in recognition of the changed conditions of fighting, they still indicate that Johnny, like the British and the Russian soldier, has the backing of the best Medical Services the world has ever known.

Chapter XIV

WHEN SWORDS WILL BE SHEATHED

IN all the preceding chapters of this volume we have discussed the present-day miracles of military medicine, the life-saving weapons which were lacking a few years ago but which doctors now possess and daily utilize. The conditions met by the wounded in this war are quite correctly compared with those of the first World War. There is, however, a danger accompanying such a comparison in that we may forget the continuous nature of the development of military medicine. If we think merely in terms of comparison between two wars, we see the past but dimly and the future not at all. We see some techniques and procedures vastly improved and find it good. We see other phases of war medicine virtually unchanged, with the doctor in these fortunately few fields able to do little more for the wounded than decades ago. Without the perspective of history, we have no way of judging either change or lack of change. And instead of finding hope in our great advances we may discover despair because, for all our growth we have yet so far to go in medicine and surgery.

We get an entirely different picture of both the present and the future, when we consider war medicine in the light of its past. Particularly do we find that the doctors of the last war, who look so weak and foolish when only their mistakes and their ignorance are considered, were actually recording just as great a series of advances as are the present-day physicians who wear the military uniform.

Consider, for example, typhoid fever, a disease once thought to be an inevitable accompaniment of every mobilization. In the Spanish-American War 14,800 men out of every 100,000 died from typhoid. By 1918, thanks to the vaccinations the Army had made compulsory since 1911, the typhoid rate was reduced to thirty-seven per 100,000, the typhoid death rate to five per 100,000. If the rate of the Spanish-American War had continued undiminished, 1918 would have seen over half a million cases, instead of a couple of hundred. Now carry the story of progress further forward. There were but two deaths from typhoid in our entire Army in 1940. In the first half of 1941, there were but three cases in a *million* and not a single death.

Similar examples could be cited for half a score of diseases, examples which conclusively demonstrate the continuity of medical advance, the building of today's "newer therapy" upon the basis of last year's (or last war's) "new method." If we have cut the pneumonia death rate to less than one-twentieth that of our 1917

Army, let us not forget that the doctors of that day could cite similar—and for that earlier time—more impressive figures of their own reduction of the death rate from smallpox, malaria, dengue, cholera, and many other diseases. Similar lessons might be drawn, *ad infinitum,* with respect to organization, surgery, sanitation, and virtually every other phase of military medicine.

Significant too, is the development in military medicine and surgery which occurred during the first World War. That conflict, like the present one, followed at least a generation of relative peace in which the main body of the medical profession had time to forget the lessons of older wars, time in which to fail to apply the newest discoveries of civil medicine to the solution of military-medical problems. It too found the problems of war surgery so different from what the memory of earlier and lesser combats had led doctors to expect that, for a time, medicine was helpless before new wounds and new diseases. It was only in 1916 that the British and French doctors of the first World War really managed to take hold of such problems as those presented by wound infection. The statistics of that war cite a sharp drop in fatalities due to infection or surgical failure occurring during the middle period of that war, a drop due to the "education" of the doctors in the first year and to the invention of new techniques and the rediscovery of old, discarded but effective ones.

Thus, if we are encouraged by the advances medicine has scored so far in this war, let us remember that many of these represent the application of the practices and discoveries of civil medicine to the problems of this conflict. The sulfa drugs, the quinine substitutes, and blood preservation were all widely used before the start of this war. Even their use for the treatment of wounds is not entirely new, since auto and industrial accidents are quite similar in many respects to war wounds. Most of the new surgical techniques have their counterparts in civil pre-war practice. The novelty or newness of our "miracles" lies in their effectiveness as compared with earlier wars, a limitation that in no way detracts from their "miraculous" nature.

But what about the experience the doctors have had during the early stages of this war? Can we not expect surgery, medicine, and chemistry to produce more miracles to match the advances of the latter half of World War I? To answer that question we must trespass on the grounds of prophecy where pitfalls are many and the bleached bones of wrong-guessers dot the way. Yet, already we find a few indications of more and more miraculous "miracles" to come.

We have told the story of our victorious fight against shock, first with direct transfusions, then with banked whole blood, then with plasma, and today with dried

plasma which may be carried anywhere, stored indefinitely and administered "on the spot" almost wherever
that may prove to be. But where do we go from there?

We may soon see the plasma fraction of blood further broken down. Dr. S. J. Cohn, a Harvard re-
searcher, has conducted extensive experiments with
human albumen, the part of blood plasma which contains about sixty-five per cent of the plasma proteins
and provides about eighty-five per cent of the osmotic
pressure—the counter shock factor—exerted by the
blood. One hundred cubic centimeters of human albumen exert the same pressure as one thousand cubic
centimeters of whole blood and may be expected to
be correspondingly effective. Thus a still smaller and
more convenient anti-shock injection is already in
sight.

Another group of researchers, working under O. H.
Wangensteen, has done much work with bovine
plasma. If the plasma of cows' blood could be utilized,
the entire problem of supply would be vastly simpli-
fied. To date, reactions to bovine plasma have run
high and the use of this blood substitute has not yet
proved practicable. Dr. Cohn, however, has been
working on a purified bovine albumen. If this should
prove acceptable both the problems of source and
concentration would be solved simultaneously. Others
are working on other blood substitutes. Drs. Taylor
and Waters have recently reported on experiments

with isinglass or fish gelatin. Harman and his associates have published a preliminary report on the use of pectin, derived from apples, as an anti-shock injection material. Just which of these, if any, are false leads and which true it is much too early to say. But the trend is well summed up by Dr. John J. Moorhead who writes, "Before World War II is won, my belief is that stored blood will be in the form of capsules or tablets and perhaps even some modifications permitting the use of animal blood already endowed to offset the prevailing organisms of the germ-infested terrain now actually world-wide."

Wound healing is a process which, naturally, concerns every military surgeon. Yet, until very recently, the best the surgeons could do was to get done with their work as fast as possible and then leave healing to nature. Now, seemingly in a confusing flood, new ideas of the nature of the body's healing mechanism have brought forth a dozen or more theories concerning wound healing. Some studies, in fact, advanced well beyond the theoretical stage and we may safely expect a rapid growth in development along these lines.

The vitamins have been looked upon as a likely source of leads in this research, since so many diseases have been shown in recent years to be the results of vitamin deficiency. Researchers have quite naturally figured that an adequacy of certain of the specialized vitamins might hasten the regrowth of cells in a wounded area. To date the most likely seem to be Vitamin B_1 or Thiamin Chloride, and Vitamin C, recently renamed Cevitamic Acid. The synthetically prepared B_1 has been found to be identical with the enzyme, secreted by the body, which governs metabolism in nerve tissue. Thus, wherever nerves are shattered, an adequate supply of B_1 in the diet will hasten recovery. Vitamin C is essential to the production of all the intercellular substances of the body and the collagen base of all fibrous tissue. The lack of Cevitamic Acid results in a tendency to hemorrhage into the wound with a consequent lag in healing. Most armies and particularly our own attempt to provide the necessary vitamins via the regular daily food ration. In the case of Vitamin C, however, it has been found that men working under great heat or exposed for long periods in a hot climate, sweat away most of the reserve of Cevitamic Acid. To make up this deficiency, our troops in these circumstances get a special ration in pill form.

Vitamin K is responsible for maintaining the level of blood prothrombin, an anti-bleeding factor. It is absorbed only in the presence of bile secretions. Thus when biliary obstructions are present, either from wounds or for other causes, a K deficiency occurs. Much experimentation is now going on to determine the best method of making up this deficiency and thus reducing the tendency of K-deficient patients to bleed profusely.

In contrast with the vitamin researches, which seek to put the body into a better functional condition for the furtherance of the healing process, there is a long tradition of search for agents that can eliminate or minimize infective organisms within the wound and thus hasten healing by removing a foreign deterrent to the natural healing process. The last war produced the famous Dakin solution and the maggot treatment. Both of these are little used today, having been replaced in favor by the sulfa drugs. A number of interesting new bactericidal or bacteriostatic drugs may yet give serious competition to the sulfonamides.

Cod liver oil is widely used in England for the treatment of infected wounds, particularly open wounds. It has been found that the oil discourages bacterial growth and simultaneously stimulates the growth of granulation tissues. But recently many doctors have swung to the theory that the effective agent in the oil is Vitamin D. For one thing, they have noticed that the raw oil is more effective than a highly purified product. And the odorous untreated oil contains more Vitamin D. They have also found that irradiation of other oils with Vitamin D increases their healing potential.

Chlorophyll, the green element in tree leaves and green vegetables, is also being tried for the treatment of infected wounds. The belief today is that it works by preventing the bacteria from digesting cell membranes. It might be said that chlorophyll starves the bacteria to death. Chlorophyll may be given by injection into the veins, by mouth, or as an irrigating fluid injected directly into the wound. It may also be used in suppositories or as an ointment. This freedom and variety of application should greatly widen its usefulness. Important too is the ease and cheapness with which the product may be prepared.

Another new drug represents the rediscovery of the potency of an herb long used by primitive savages. Barberry has been found to contain an active agent, berberine, which is effective in killing erysipelas streptococci. The drug is dangerous when administered intravenously and this may limit its usefulness.

Apple diets are a world-wide remedy for infant diarrhea. Recent research shows the effective agent to be pectin, which both inhibits bacterial growth and promotes granulation. Interestingly, this is the same material being tried out as a blood substitute. It too should be easy and cheap to prepare.

One of the strangest new proposals calls for the use of finely powdered silicon as a healing agent for wounds and ulcers. This suggestion seems all the more startling when we remember that the stonecutters' disease, silicosis, gets its name from the fine silicon dust which causes lung tissues to become fibrous and hence useless. Yet this very quality, so deadly in the lungs, is the one sought in the current proposals. For in a wound, the early formation of tissue fibers is exactly what is wanted. Here again, folk medicine has anticipated a scientific discovery, for the Appalachian mountaineers have long had a tradition that eating sand, *i.e., silicon*, will cause bleeding ulcers to disappear. At the University of Cincinnati, for a number of years studies have been under way on the use of silicon powders for both ulcers and bleeding tumors. The favorable results there obtained have led some authorities to list this as one of the possible new methods of encouraging wound healing.

Quite as startling, to the layman at least, are two new germ killers known as Gramicidin and Penecillin. Both are brewed by bacteria that live in soil and both are far stronger in their bactericidal action than the sulfa drugs. Two things have, until recently, delayed widespread experimentation with these drugs. First was the fact that they were found to destroy the red blood cells of the patient when injected into the blood stream. This has been overcome by direct application to the wound, though such application is probably limited in its sphere to wounds of certain types only. The other is the difficulty of extracting the drugs, which are extremely expensive and available today only for research and then only in minute quantities.

Next to the United States, the Soviet Union has

shown more interest in the development of new healing agents than any other country. Unfortunately, the
medical liaison between ourselves and our ally has
always been of a most sketchy nature and, often
enough, it has been found that the scientists of both
countries have been pursuing the same line of research
independently. Under the stimulus of the war, no
doubt, a closer alliance between researchers will probably be built up, as it has already been built, to a
marked degree, between British and Soviet scientists.

Much of the Russian research in recent years has
been devoted to long-term projects such as the extended investigations into the domain of longevity
conducted by the Soviet Academician A. A. Bogomelets and his associates. Today, however, some of the
discoveries of this group are paying an unexpected
dividend to the youngsters among the Red Army's
wounded. It has long been known that one of the characteristics of age has been a slowing-up of the ability
of tissues to heal after injury. According to Bogomelets
the normal span of human life could be extended to
as much as 150 years, if we could prevent cell-thick-
ening, sclerotic changes from occurring in the connec-
tive tissues of the body. Early in 1941, the Russians
developed what they call an "anti-reticular cytotoxic
serum," which they believe has the power to change
the properties of the protoplasm of aging cells, making
them resemble the protoplasm of a young organism.

The serum produced highly gratifying results in the treatment of sclerosis and in the early stages of high blood pressure.

With the Nazi attack on the Soviet Union, the problems of retarding aging became, for the moment, far less important to Russian science than those of healing the wounded. Bogomelets and his associates therefore switched their research towards a direct application of the new serum to the acceleration of wound healing. Early reports from the Red Army hospitals indicate that the serum is particularly useful in the treatment of difficult knitting fractures caused by shell splinters and for ulcers and other slow-healing wounds.

In respect to all new drugs, the United States enjoys one advantage which was not ours during the last war. Just how important this advantage has already proved to be is demonstrated by the contrast with Britain. Unlike this country, the English possess no highly developed drug and biological industry. The Germans were the first to develop the production of drugs along the lines of large industry. At the turn of the century, while other countries still relied upon individual pharmacists and small chemical houses, the German dye trust gathered to itself all the elements of large-scale drug production. It was not content to rest on its ability to synthesize drugs from the coal-tar derivatives of its dye business, but spent vast sums on its own research laboratories and the subsidization of hospital and university research. Thus, by 1914, it had virtually complete control of the major world drug markets. In the United States, the dislocations brought on by the first World War led to the Americanization of German drug patents and the rapid development of our own drug industry.

In Britain, however, the post war decades saw a quick return to the old habit of relying upon German and Swiss imports for most of the synthetic drugs and anaesthetics. England today relies in large measure upon Lend-Lease supplies from this country. The attempt to build such an industry, after World War II began, was hampered by the lack of trained workers. There was, for instance, not a single trained barbiturate chemist in all Great Britain at the time the war started, in contrast to the more than twenty full-time research workers maintained by the Germans in this field.

By way of contrast, the commercial drug industry in this country grew by leaps and bounds in the years since 1918. In part this has been the result of our curious propensity for self-medication, Americans being the easiest people in the world to whom to sell a new drug, hormone, vitamin, or just plain cure-all. Yet our ingestion of countless pills we did not need and countless others that made us healthier, has served to supply the funds which have maintained the great private research laboratories. With the laboratories maintained by semi-public institutions, universities, and the various governmental bodies, these have served to build up our reservoir of trained chemical and biological workers. Thus, we are today in a position to put any new discovery quickly into use, reducing its synthesis or extraction to the low-cost level of a mass-production procedure.

The highly integrated nature of our food industry, which once made us the only nation to suffer from vitamin deficiency because its bread was too refined, today is producing nutritional miracles which minimize the injury and hasten the repair of wounds. Our soldiers are healthier than they have ever been before and they are being kept healthy by scientific planning. Much of the credit for the maintenance of their health under the adverse conditions of warfare must go to the Army's Subsistence Research Laboratory where, for ten years, a small group known as the "Guinea Pig Club" has been developing new Army rations and turning them over to food-processing concerns for production.

The latest prize package to emerge from the Chicago laboratories is known as Food Ration K, a far cry from the hardtack that once constituted the only food of soldiers on difficult missions away from regular mess sources. Ration K comes in a heat-and-cold-proof box measuring only six-by-six-by-four inches, yet it provides a surprisingly tasty and varied menu. Its three meals include a breakfast of compressed graham crackers, veal luncheon meat, fruit bar, malted milk dextrose tablets, soluble coffee, sugar, chewing gum, and four cigarettes. Its dinner omits the fruit bar and supplies, instead, a powdered bouillon. Supper consists of biscuits, cheese, fruit-juice powder, a chocolate bar, sugar, chewing gum, and cigarettes. The K Ration was recently tried by mountain troops on the Mount Rainier glaciers and on the desert at Indio, California, where the temperature ranges around 122 degrees in the shade. In both trials the troops came through in fine shape, despite strenuous labors simulating actual battle conditions.

On a larger scale, our food industries have worked numerous miracles, making it possible to beat the shipping shortage without cutting down on the quality of food. Lend-Lease supplies now include millions of cases of dehydrated eggs, meats, and vegetables, shorn of their water and thus of their bulk, but retaining both tastiness and food values. A new "de-bone-ing" procedure now permits more than twice as much Chicago beef to ship in a single hold than could have been placed there before. Yet, for all this, the advances in food preparation which have reached the stage of actual application in the last two years are but the forerunners of further advances that are just now coming out of the laboratory. There is not the slightest question but that this war's soldiers will be better able to resist disease and to repair their wounds than any body of men who ever fought before.

Surgery, too, has some new tricks up its sleeves. It is not too likely that revolutionary new types of operations will come out of this war's surgery, for almost every region and organ of the body has long been subject to surgical intervention. The trends in the newer surgery seem to be concerned more with the development of instruments and materials to facilitate operations or hasten post-operative recovery. Here, as elsewhere in our complicated lives, the shift has been from purely mechanical devices to instruments utilizing or modifying discoveries in radio and electronic science. Surgeons in an earlier era were among the most prolific of inventors, filling the catalogues of the instrument makers with an infinite variety of forceps, scalpels, splints, and optical devices, all designed to aid the specialist in seeing the site of his operation and cutting or sewing with the greatest speed and the least strain to both surgeon and patient. Such instruments still appear, one of the newest being an improved surgical needle, a veritable automatic body-stitcher, put out appropriately enough by the Singer Sewing Machine people.

But more and more of the newer devices utilize electrical rather than merely mechanical principles. The electroencephalograph permits the doctor to localize brain troubles with fair accuracy, although its development and particularly our understanding of its potentialities is still in its infancy. This instrument locates and measures the extremely minute electrical impulses set up by brain processes and distinguishes between normal and diseased "brain waves." The electric foreign-body locator and the electro-cautery knife have already been discussed in some detail in earlier chapters. The electrocardiograph is widely used for the study of heart action. Yet these infinitely precise and amazingly complex instruments are but the forerunners of devices to come which will utilize electricity either to analyze and diagnose bodily conditions or to stimulate the body's reparative mechanisms.

In recent years, the sterilizing properties of ultra-violet light have come in for much attention. Such lights were first used industrially, to insure sterility for public washrooms and to sterilize all sorts of industrial products from cold creams to breakfast foods. For such purposes the lights are most convenient, since a short exposure provides a high degree of sterilization. In factories, products flowing by on belt conveyors, on their way from one process to the next, can be sterilized by passage through a metal tunnel lighted by a battery of ultra-violet lamps. Naturally, physicians have been quick to pick up this development and apply it to the ever-present problem of keeping their operating theaters surgically clean. Many a hospital today uses such lamps to shine protectively over instruments and surgical swabs during an operation. Some doctors advocate the use of these lights to sterilize hands and garments at the entrances to operating rooms.

But just recently Dr. Miley has announced what is perhaps the first direct surgical use of ultra-violet light in a report on 151 patients suffering from acute pyogenic infections. These cases, with blood poisoned by pus-forming bacteria, had failed to recover from peritonitis, lobar pneumonia, poisoned wounds, or other manifestations of the infection, even when treated with sulfa drugs. Dr. Miley and his associates at Hahnemann Medical College in Philadelphia drew off some of the patients' blood, exposed it to ultra-violet light for about ten seconds, and immediately re-injected it.

Of 35 acute cases treated in the early stages, all recovered. Of 61 advanced cases, all but one survived. And 23 out of 55 who would once have been counted as hopeless, patients who were already in advanced stages of coma, were brought back to life by the simple procedure. If future experimentation bears out the physicians' seemingly well-founded hopes in this method, medicine will have found a new, speedy, and almost completely painless way of fighting war wound infections; something more effective in its special field, than even the sulfa drugs we have today.

After the last war, nerve surgeons worked out many remarkable operations for the suturing of severed nerves. Often a severe wound left a gap in a major nerve of three inches or more. Taking advantage of the devious courses followed by nerves, which make them often substantially longer than the distance they actually traverse from point to point, these surgeons would virtually dig out the remaining nerve tissues at either end of the destroyed areas and replace them into newly cut beds. The more direct line of the new bed would permit a juxtaposition of the nerve ends and, often enough, these ends would grow together and nerve function be restored. This was, however, a most difficult and tortuous procedure, for which skilled surgeons could hardly be spared under the stress of active warfare. In England, recently, two British surgeons have reported on a new method of achieving a reconnection of severed nerves that may provide the same—and possibly even better—results without the strain on doctor and patient. These doctors noted that nerves have the ability to regenerate to a high degree, extending their growth along their axis. They sought therefore to channelize this growth so that the severed nerve ends would, as it were, find each other. To do so, they prepared a bed between the two ends of the injured nerve, filling it with dried blood plasma. Much to their satisfaction they found that growth proceeded down this path, until the meeting ends fused into a new, functioning nerve. It is too early, as yet, to say whether this procedure will prove valuable in practice, but if it should, much of the crippling effect of wound injuries may in the future be eliminated.

Some of the things the more ambitious surgeons talk about, in their more loquacious moments, are enough to lead the lay listener to think himself the victim of a bit of medical leg-pulling. Yet often enough, the seemingly ridiculous forecast proves incorrect only in so far as it turns out to have been too conservative. Such might be the reaction to one doctor's serious statement that all the preconditions are now available for the invention of a surgical glue, by which wounds could be pasted up instead of sewn or left to nature to be seamed anew. Yet, investigation discloses that much serious and expensive research is under way along these lines, both in this country and abroad, although surgical suture-makers have not yet thought it necessary to curtail production in anticipation of the realization of this dream.

In fighting disease new developments, placing a comparable tax on the credulity of the layman, are likewise just barely offstage. There is not the slightest doubt that chemotherapy will make advances in the next few years that will make the miracles of the sulfa drugs seem tame. Certainly our new understanding of the mechanism of the chemical and physical processes of bacteria permits a logical approach to the search for new chemo-therapeutic agents for the first time to replace hit-or-miss experimentation. But chemotherapy, which has seemed to some to have decreased the importance of research on immunization and specific serums for fighting specific disease, may yet lead us back to a new and higher level of serum treatment. For the better understanding of the mechanisms of bacterial action within the body, which the studies of the sulfa investigators have given us, has now stimulated the search for artificial manufactured serums.

At the California School of Technology, two biochemists, Linus Pauling and Dan Campbell, have actually succeeded in creating artificial antibodies, synthetic test-tube creations that duplicate the action of the disease-fighting substances thrown up by the blood stream to destroy invading bacteria. The Pauling-Campbell theory is that natural antibodies are rearranged molecules of the blood proteins known as serum globulin. When bacteria or poison cells approach a globulin molecule in the body, according to this theory, the globulin unit changes its shape and assumes a new structure so that it can combine with the invading molecule and neutralize it. After the disease has been overcome, these changed molecules or antibodies remain in the blood stream ready to attack later invaders. The body thus enjoys "immunity."

Up to now the miracle of immunization lay in our ability to transfer antibodies from one living animal to another, either from human to human or from horses or other animals. Moreover, we could transfer small quantities of these antibodies and use them to stimulate the formation of such additional substances within the body of the recipient. As if this was not miracle enough, Pauling and Campbell have now succeeded in performing the miracle in the laboratory. To date they have made antibodies of only limited applicability against some chemical poisons and the bacteria of one strain of pneumonia. But they have proved that it can be done and opened the door to newer, simpler methods of *manufacturing* immunity against disease.

The examples of progress in medicine which have been here cited are but a small fraction of the developments actually under way today. Hundreds of published reports open other, equally exciting vistas. And undoubtedly much of the most promising work has not as yet received any mention even in the abstruse and virtually unreadable journals used by technical workers for the exchange of their new-found information.

Under the stimulus of the war, which both increases our urgent need for these advances and provides the medical profession and its associate technologists with the practice that accelerates development, we may confidently count upon taking many another sting out of the wounds of war before our swords are again sheathed. But what about the future? When the war finally ends, a shattered, impoverished, undernourished world will certainly need all the medicine and the best medicine that modern science can supply. Will it get it—will medical progress be as equal to the differing but no less exacting needs of peace as it is proving to be in war?

The answer is simple and it is the same answer that applies to every other question affecting our lives today. It all depends on who wins the war. For scientific progress, including that of medicine, is not to be dissociated from the rest of our world. Nazism lays its heavy hand on science with the same ruthless efficiency with which it attacks all the other values which free men hold dear. This may not be apparent at first glance, for the very sinews of the Hitler machine have come out of the highly developed scientific laboratories of the German dye and steel and chemical trusts. Yet, if we look closer, we can see a progressive deterioration of all German science in the years since Hitler came to power.

This trend made itself apparent in German medicine almost immediately, for many of Germany's foremost research workers were, like Ehrlich, Jews. And many another German scientist, though lacking nothing in Aryan ancestry, could not stomach the rule of the gauleiters and ended his career either in exile or in a concentration camp. In science, as everywhere else, the Hitler revolution opened the way wide for the advance of the mediocre over men of learning and ability. More and more, the new "scientists" of Germany tended to be either professional Nazi hacks or those who fooled themselves into thinking they might buy the right to research by being "non-political." Even that hope proved a will-o'-the-wisp, for Nazism cannot tolerate free research just as it cannot·permit free thought; both may lead to conclusions against the interest of the Nazi state.

Thus German medicine, like all German science, has had to adapt itself to the distortions necessitated by Nazi doctrine. A single example will suffice to show to what realms of nonsense such adaptation may lead. The good Nazi doctor cannot save his Aryan, superman patient's life with the blood of a non-Aryan. German prisoners of war have actually, incredible as it may seem, refused transfusions in Britain because they could not be certain that the blood they received would be of the proper Teutonic extraction.

Though in its more pervasive manifestations, Nazi doctrine runs counter to all scientific thought, some have thought that, at least in the field of practice, the Nazis would be among the first to utilize science to the fullest. Yet time after incredible time, they have shackled themselves, even hurt their war effort, by resolving the conflict between science and Nazism in favor of the latter. Common sense and common science would tell them that the spread of infectious disease anywhere in Europe would endanger their own health. Yet they have calmly permitted plagues to decimate the population of conquered areas throughout Europe, despite the danger to themselves, in their haste to make room for the master race. Nazi science, in medicine as in war, it becomes increasingly clear, is the science of death. If we lose the war, if we permit ourselves to do so, we cannot expect anything better than the "science" that now distinguishes the Poles from their pigs only to favor the pigs.

But winning the war alongside of the free people of all the world . . . what then? Again we must judge the future in the light of the past. Just as after the last war, civil medicine will no doubt advance because of the experience our doctors will have gained in war. The advance should, in fact, be more marked this time, for war differs less than it did in the past from the hazards of peace. Our new knowledge of war medicine will prove immeasurably helpful in the development of aviation, in fighting industrial accidents, in opening up the tropics to human habitation at a high standard of living. The organized, co-operative work of our doctors (necessitated both by the needs of military discipline and by the pressure of civil work on the physicians who remain at home) should teach our doctors new ways of working, new ways of bringing medicine to the people, of making the advances of medical science less a matter of having the price than they have ever been in the past. The words socialized medicine have become fighting words among physicians in recent years. Yet war medicine in the army is completely socialized. And at home, it assumes new co-operative forms under our very eyes. Just how medicine will be organized after the war, we cannot say. But certainly it will not pass up the goal of reaching more people which the war has forced it to achieve.

Our younger doctors, the ones who would have waited for patients throughout the 1940's, will return from this war, as their fathers did from the last, with two decades of experience compressed into a few years. Our medical education facilities will probably not again be allowed to contract after this war, not if we learn anything from the present shortage of physicians we are now experiencing. International exchange of medical technique and information should reach a new high level in a post-war world, unless again we prove unequal to our opportunities. Certainly the British, the Russians, the Chinese, and ourselves should now be learning much we never knew before of how to co-operate in advancing the science of human health. Our medical men, engaged today in doing more for the soldier than they ever were able to do before, can thus look forward to specialized goals for their science which should make a victorious peace even more attractive to them than to any of the rest of us.